FREEDOM FROM ECZEMA

Eliminate Acne, Eczema, and Candidiasis –
Find Out How ...

Devi S. Nambudripad,
M.D., D.C., L.Ac., Ph.D. (Acu.)

Author of the book series
"*Say Good-bye to ...*" and **"*Freedom From ...*"**

This information has already revolutionized
THE PRACTICE OF MEDICINE

The doctor of the future will give no medicine,
But will interest his patients
In the care of the human frame, in diet,
And in the cause and prevention of disease.
Thomas A. Edison

DELTA PUBLISHING COMPANY
6714 Beach Blvd., Buena Park, CA 90621
(888) 890-0670, (714) 523-8900 Fax: (714) 523-3068
Web site: www.naet.com

D1603902

DEDICATION

This book is dedicated to
patients, who suffer from eczema and other skin disorders
and any one wishing to get well through NAET®

First Edition, 2008
Copyright © 2008 by
Devi S. Nambudripad, M.D., D.C., L.Ac., Ph.D. (Acu.)
Buena Park, California
All rights reserved.

Library of Congress Control No: 2007932102

ISBN: 978-1-934523-01-8

Printed in the U.S.A.

Contents

CHAPTER 1
WHAT ARE COMMON SKIN DISORDERS?
Understanding Symptoms and Causes

CHAPTER 2
WHAT TYPES OF ALLERGIES TRIGGER SKIN DISORDERS?
Taking a Closer Look: Categories of Allergens

CHAPTER 3
HOW ARE ALLERGY-RELATEDSKIN DISORDERS DIAGNOSED?
Finding the Underlying Problem

CHAPTER 4
HOW ARE ALLERGY-RELATED SKIN DISORDERS TREATED?
Eliminating the Problem

CHAPTER 5
A COLLECTION OF NAET® SUCCESS STORIES
Freedom from Allergies!

Acknowledgments

I am deeply grateful to my husband, Kris Nambudripad, for his encouragement and assistance in my schooling, and later in the formulation of this project. Without his cooperation in researching content, revising manuscripts, word processing and proofreading, it is doubtful whether this book would have ever been completed.

My sincere thanks also go to the many clients who have entrusted their care to me, for without them I would have had no case studies, no feedback, and certainly no extensive source of personal research upon which to base this book.

I am also deeply grateful to Helen Tanner, Karen Watts, Margaret Brazil, Jennifer Bentley, Helene Singer, Lettie Vipond, Shirley Reason, Toby Weiss, Terri Weiss, Amy Clute, Rosemary Depau, Margaret Davies, Barbara Cortez, Devon Cesmat, Michael Magrutch, Jeanne Elston, Jeanne Soriano, Neeta P., Connie Kilona, Nancy M., and Karen Tuckerman, to name a few among many of my devoted patients, for believing in me to be treated with NAET®. I am grateful to these enthusiastic patients who helped me develop effective NAET® for various health problems, including skin disorders, by supporting my theory and helping me to conduct the ongoing detective work on them.

I also have to express my thanks to my son, Roy, who assisted me in many ways in writing this book. He suffered from atopic dermatitis, contact dermatitis, itching, and acne (especially on his back) whenever he consumed or contacted allergic products, until he eliminated all of his known allergies through NAET® treatment.

I would like to extend my thanks to Robert Prince, M.D., Laurie Teitelbaum, M.S., and many of my associates who wish to remain anonymous for assisting me with this work, and Mr. Roy at Delta Publishing for his printing expertise. I am deeply grateful for my professional training and the knowledge and skills acquired in classes and seminars on chiropractic and kinesiology at the Southern California University, in Whittier, California; the California Acupuncture College in Los Angeles; SAMRA University of Oriental Medicine, Los Angeles; University of Health Sciences, School of Medicine, Antigua; and the clinical experience received at the clinics associated with these colleges.

My special thanks also go to Mala Moosad, N.D., R.N., L.Ac., Ph.D., and Mohan Moosad, M.S., N.D., L.Ac, who supported and stood by me since the very beginning, from my NAET® discovery through our ongoing research. Mala and Mohan also helped me immensely by taking over my work at the clinic so that I could complete the book. I also would like to acknowledge my thanks to my dear mother for continuing to nourish me emotionally and nutritionally since childhood. My heartfelt thanks also go to Margaret Wu and Barbara Cesmat, NAET® practitioners, who have dedicated their time to help desperate allergy sufferers by assisting me in many ways to promote my mission of making NAET® available to everyone who needs help around the world. I would also like to acknowledge my everlasting thanks to my office manager, Janna Gossen, who has worked with me from the first day of my practice over two decades ago, and all of the other staff members and NAET® practitioners who support me and stand with me to help more victims of allergies find health through NAET®.

I would like to remember the late Dr. Richard F. Farquhar at Farquhar Chiropractic Clinic in Bellflower, California. I was a student of chiropractic and acupuncture when I was doing preceptorship with him. When I told him about my NAET® discovery, he tried the treatment on himself and was amazed with the results. Then he encouraged me to practice NAET® with acupuncture on all of his patients. Because of his generosity, I had the opportunity to treat hundreds of patients soon after I discovered NAET®.

I am so delighted to express my sincere thanks to the Los Angeles College of Chiropractic for teaching different branches of holistic medicine (such as kinesiology and sacro-occipital techniques) along with chiropractic, and providing the students with a sound knowledge of nutrition. Because of that, I was able to combine the art of kinesiology, chiropractic, and nutrition, along with acupuncture/acupressure, to develop NAET®. California Acupuncture College also taught me a few lessons in kinesiology along with the art and science of acupuncture. I do not have enough words to express my heartfelt thanks and appreciation to California Acupuncture State Board for supporting NAET® from the beginning, permitting me to teach other licensed acupuncturists, by instantly making me a CEU provider soon after I discovered NAET®. Perhaps the California Acupuncture State Board will never know how much they have helped humanity by validating my new technique and allowing me to share the treatment method with other practitioners and, through them, to the countless number of patients who now live a normal life. I am forever indebted to acupuncture and Oriental medicine. Without this knowledge, I, myself, would still be living in pain. Thank you for allowing me to share my experience with the world!

I also extend my sincere appreciation and thanks to my medical school professors for willing to part with their knowledge and help us become great physicians. I would like to extend my sincere thanks to these great teachers especially to my medical school mentors and professors from Antigua and California, and the staff of the respective hospitals where I did my clinicals. Without their guidance and teaching, I doubt whether I could have completed the medical school.

All of my mentors from all of the professional schools I attended have helped me to grow immensely at all levels. They are also indirectly responsible for the improvement of my personal health as well as the health of my family, patients, and other NAET® practitioners as well as their countless patients.

Many of my professors, doctors of Western and Oriental medicine, chiropractic, and kinesiology, as well as nutritionists, were willing to give of themselves by teaching and committing personal time, through interviews, to help me complete this book. I will always be eternally grateful to them. They demonstrated the highest ideals of the medical profession.

Devi S. Nambudripad, M.D., D.C., L.Ac., Ph.D. (Acu.)

Preface

Since childhood I suffered from a multitude of health problems. Because of this prolonged and firsthand experience with ill health, it is no wonder that I became focused on health-related problems, particularly those related to allergies; this, in turn, resulted in my natural inclination to pursue medicine as a profession. I began specializing in the treatment of the allergic patient, using methods I learned through an intensive study of Oriental medicine, combined with the more traditional Western methods learned from various Western medical schools that I had attended. During my studies and early practice as an allergist, while using eclectic methods of allergy treatments, I discovered a technique that eliminated most of my health problems. *Nambudripad's Allergy Elimination Techniques (NAET®)*, which has become the focus of my practice, is an integration of the relevant techniques from the various fields I studied, combined with my own discoveries.

Except for avoidance, which leads to deprivation and frustration, there is no known successful method of treatment for food allergies using Western medicine. Each of the disciplines I studied had provided bits of knowledge that I used in developing NAET®, a new treatment that permanently eliminates allergies, and is now known throughout the world. As an infant, living in India, I had severe infantile eczema, which lasted until I was seven or eight years old. I was given Western medicine and Ayurvedic herbal medicine without a break. (Ayurveda is the traditional Indian system of medicine based largely on herbs and naturopathy.) Western medicine did not help me much. While I was taking the herbal medicines, my symptoms were under control, but whenever I stopped taking the herbs, my eczema recurred. When I was eight

years old, one of the herbal doctors told my parents to feed me
only white rice cooked with a special herb formula. The ingredients of this herbal blend and the action of each herb are given in
detail in Chapter 4 (see "Rice-Detox Diet").

This special diet helped me a great deal. The herbalist seemed
to know what he was doing. These herbs were selected from a regular kitchen shelf to create the special formula, yet the herbal blend
was a powerful cleanser for the body. Through this special diet, my
body was able to eliminate the toxins I produced daily, and in a few
months my eczema cleared up. The only drawback was that I had
to be on this diet constantly. As I was growing up, I began cheating
every so often by going on and off of this diet. If I missed one day,
I suffered the consequences; so my parents made sure that I stayed
on it faithfully. Unfortunately, my good health did not last. I began to experience symptoms of arthritis. On certain days, all of my
joints ached. The pain became so severe that I often had to stay in
bed for several days. Atopic dermatitis often occurs together with
other atopic diseases (i.e., diseases commonly caused by allergies),
such as angioneurotic edema, asthma, arthritis, chronic bronchitis,
conjunctivitis, migraines, sinusitis, etc. While growing up I suffered
from all of these problems.

Infantile eczema and atopic eczema are often familial (i.e.,
they tend to occur in family members), and can be chronic. The
symptoms can increase or disappear over time. Whenever I ate the
white rice cooked with herbs, I felt better. Consequently, I started
liking white rice more and more. It became a staple diet for me.

While I was on this strict diet, I was able to continue with my
education. I completed my training in nursing, and soon after (in
1976) I married and relocated to Los Angeles. My husband had been
suffering from some health problems, and he was following a strict
diet under the supervision of a nutritionist. I became more health-
conscious, and tried to change my eating habits by adding into my
diet more fruits, vegetables, whole grain products and complex car-

bohydrates, under the advice of the same nutritionist. All of a sudden, I became very ill, with bronchitis and pneumonia, and then my arthritis and eczema returned. Symptoms continued to multiply: I suffered from insomnia, clinical depression, constant sinusitis, and frequent migraine headaches. I felt extremely tired all the time, but remained wide awake when I went to bed. I had no idea then that I was allergic to all essential nutrients.

During the next few years, I tried many different antibiotics and other mediciations, I changed doctors, and I consulted more nutritionists. All of the medications, vitamins, and herbs that I took made me more sick, and eating good, wholesome foods made me worse. I was nauseated all the time. Every inch of my body ached and felt like a train had run over me, all of the time. No one knew the source of my pain and discomfort. All laboratory reports returned normal, except the blood platelet counts which remained slightly high for a long time (around 500,000 per microliter; normal is between 130,000-400,000 per microliter). None of my physicians thought that this platelet elevation was significant enough to produce the pain and other symptoms that I was experiencing. I had to learn to live with the pain. My husband was taking one Aspirin® each day as a preventive measure (to thin the blood), as suggested by his family physician. One day I thought probably the Aspirin® might help reduce my platelets too. Although I could not find any information to support my belief, I decided to take Aspirin®, and for the first time in years I felt relief from my general bodyache. Relief lasted for only an hour, then my pains returned. I began taking more and more Aspirin® to relieve the pain for longer periods of time. I continued to take large doses of Aspirin® daily until the summer of 1984. By then I had discovered NAET®, and eliminated most of my allergies, bodyache, and fibromyalgia. Since food allergies had been causing my aches and pains, I no longer needed Aspirin® for pain relief. When I completed treatments for most of my food allergies, my platelet counts decreased and maintained around 410,000 per microliter. Since then, I have observed that most of my patients with aches and pains also had laboratory tests that showed high blood platelet counts.

In 1981, I started training at the Los Angeles College of Chiropractic. By then, I had been fighting chronic bronchitis for two years. My nutrition teacher at the college advised me to go on a juice diet. In two days, I had severe laryngitis, my bronchitis got worse, and I developed a fever of 104 degrees Fahrenheit. She said I was going through a healing crisis. In the southern part of India where I come from, when a person is sick with a common cold or fever, cooked soft rice is the prescribed food. So, I stayed home for three days, ate cooked soft white rice, and appeared to partially recover from that episode. When I returned to college, we had a guest speaker who was an acupuncturist. I was sitting in a corner of the classroom, coughing frequently. He watched me awhile and commented that I was suffering from an *attack of wind/heat* (Chinese medical term for the common cold). At the time, I did not understand what he meant. He explained a few things about acupuncture, then gave me a quick treatment using acupressure. His treatments made me feel very good and, to my surprise, I stopped coughing.

After the class was over, I asked the guest speaker for information about an acupuncture college, called the school the same day, and enrolled for classes. The very first class, entitled *Touch for Health,* was on acupressure. On the first day my instructor taught Muscle Response Testing (MRT) to detect food allergies. By then, my cough had returned. The teacher noticed my chronic, raspy cough; suspecting that I was suffering from food allergies, he tested me for various allergies to food items through MRT. I reacted to almost everything except white rice and broccoli. He suggested that I might do better if I ate only white rice and broccoli, exclusively, for a few days. (I suddenly had flashbacks to age eight when I was put on that white rice diet.)

By that time I had been examined and treated by many doctors, including neurologists, cardiologists, psychologists, psychiatrists, nutritionists, and herbalists, but none had suspected food allergies as a cause of my chronic ill health. I was excited by this new possibility. I was willing to try anything to feel better. I followed my teacher's advice and ate white rice and broccoli exclusively. Within one week, my bronchitis cleared up, my headaches became infrequent and less intense, my joint pains eased, and my back pain ceased. My thinking and concentration became more clear. My depression (that had lasted two years) disappeared. The insomnia disappeared. My general bodyaches cleared. My skin began to heal, but it did not become completely clear until after I was treated with NAET® for most food groups. For the first time in my life, I experienced pain-free days without the help of Aspirin®. It was a delight for me to go to bed without pain and wake up in the morning without pain.

After a week on a restricted diet, I tried eating some other foods, but my symptoms returned. I began eating only white rice and broccoli again. I could not eat salads, fruits, or vegetables, because (as I eventually discovered) I was very allergic to vitamin C; whole grain products because they contained B-complex; fruits, honey or any products made from sugars because I was very allergic to sugar; milk or milk products because I was very allergic to calcium; fish groups because I was allergic to vitamin A; and egg products because they caused skin problems. I was allergic to all types of dried beans, including soybeans, which gave me severe joint pains and backaches. Most spices, especially in the pepper family, gave me arthritis and migraines. Almost all fabrics, except silk, gave me itching problems, joint pain, and caused extreme tiredness. My teacher at the acupuncture college confirmed my doubts: I was simply allergic to everything under the sun, including the sun by radiation.

It seemed that I was allergic to everything except white rice, broccoli, silk and Aspirin®. What a combination! At least I was lucky to have a few non-allergic items. In my practice, I now see many less fortunate patients, who have allergies to everything imaginable. Most of them were living the equivalent of being in a bubble before they were treated with NAET®.

In 1980, after three miscarriages, my son was born, and I was overjoyed. However, since birth he too suffered from numerous allergies, including severe infantile eczema, atopic eczema, cradle cap, diaper rash, whole-body rash, and frequent hives. (In 1984 he was treated with NAET® for his allergies to milk, grains, vitamin C mix, vegetables, fruits, sugar, oils, butter, cotton, chlorine bleach, and insects, and his skin became normal.)

From 1980 through most of 1983, I continued to live on the restricted diet of white rice and broccoli for three and a half years. On Friday, November 23, 1983, I came home from school and found that I did not have any more cooked rice. I started to cook more rice, and happened to eat a few pieces of carrot while I was waiting for the rice to finish cooking. In just a few minutes, I felt tired, lethargic, and like I was going to pass out. I inserted acupuncture needles to prevent me from fainting. During the acupuncture treatment, I fell asleep, and the carrots were still in my hand. At around 2:00 p.m., after the acupuncture treatment (and a restful nap during the needling period), I woke up and experienced a unique feeling. I had never felt quite that way after similar acupuncture treatments in the past. I realized that I still had some carrot in my hand, and that I had also been lying on some of the carrot. I knew that some of the needles were supposed to help circulate the electrical energy and balance the body. (The balancing treatment process clears energy blockages. I had studied this concept at school.)

I had asked my husband, who had been assisting me in the treatment process, to test me for carrots again. My MRT remained strong, indicating that I was no longer allergic to carrots. After putting "two and two together," I understood that the carrot's energy field had interacted with my own energy field, and my brain had

learned to accept as harmless what had once been a deadly poison. The two energy fields no longer clashed. This was an amazing NEW DISCOVERY. Subsequent MRT for carrots confirmed
that something phenomenal had happened. We repeated testing
every hour for the rest of that day. I continued eating carrots the
next day without any allergic reaction. This confirmed the result.
My central nervous system had learned a different response to the
stimulus, and I was no longer reactive to it. In some mysterious
way, the treatment had reprogrammed my brain.

What followed was a series of experiments in treating my allergies and my family members' allergies. These experiments began with an increased understanding of the connection between my
body and the carrot. While studying at the acupuncture college that
semester, I attended a class in *Electromagnetic Fields and Acupuncture*. The class taught that every object on earth, whether living or
nonliving, possesses a surrounding electromagnetic energy field.
Earth has its own energy field. Every object is attracted to Earth.
Every object is also attracted to one another. All of these different
energies can attract or repel, depending upon their energy differences. My body and the carrot each had its own electromagnetic field.

I realized that physical contact with the allergen during NAET®
treatment produces the necessary immune mediators (antidotes)
to neutralize the allergen's adverse reaction. This produces a totally new, permanent and irreversible response to the allergen. It
is possible, through stimulation of the appropriate points of the
acupuncture meridians (which have direct correspondence with
the brain), to reprogram the brain.

I cured most of my allergies and allergy-based health problems, including my eczema, within a year. Later, I extended this
to my patients who suffered from a multitude of symptoms that
arose from allergies. In every case, allergies were "cleared out,"
never to return.

My amazing recovery and return to health has since been replicated in thousands of my patients, who were treated with NAET® for a wide variety of allergens and allergy-related disorders. The procedure is no longer experimental or of questionable value. NAET® is a now a proven treatment method, and is used by more than 10,000 health care professionals around the world. The success of the NAET® procedure confirms that many illnesses indeed result from allergies.

The more extensively I studied the subject of allergies, the more I found it to be truly fascinating, yet highly complex. In the last few years, a separate area of medical study has emerged based on growing acceptance of the idea that food allergies can cause multiple physiological problems. However, this field does not have the recognition that it deserves. Part of the problem is that the Western medicine approach for evaluating allergies is cumbersome. No refined laboratory test is available to detect all posible hypersensitivities, intolerances, and true allergies. Using only Western allergy testing methods, most allergies, sensitivities, and reactions go unnoticed, and the symptoms arising from such uncharted reactions remain unsolved. The result is that unidentified allergic reactions are causing a myriad of unsolved health problems, including various skin disorders that are labeled as incurable. Using only the Western medicine approach, research has been limited by testing methodologies and the common association between allergens and allergic manifestations. However, incorporating the Oriental medicine approach, NAET® can determine which specific allergen is causing even the most mild energy disturbance in the body.

Anyone with a skin disorder should have a complete physical examination and evaluation to rule out non-allergic factors that may be involved. However, if the findings of all tests are negative, then "an allergy" is likely to be the root cause of symptoms. If that is the case, it is best to find an NAET® Specialist, who can find the cause of the allergy and eliminate the problem.

I have published several books on NAET® and allergies. In each of those books, I have focused on identifying the causative agent via Oriental medicine testing procedures, and then managing allergies, allergic reactions, or allergy-related health disorders through NAET®. Most of my books carry descriptions of meridians, testing procedures, and some self-help tips. The book, "*Say Good-bye to Illness*" is the melting pot for various health-related information in a very concise format. In the companion books, I have focused on particular health issues, because several of my patients had requested that I write a book focused on their particular health issue. The reason for such requests, they said, was because they regained their health through NAET® but were unable to explain it adequately to their friends and colleagues who had similar health problems. They were aware that NAET® could help with a wide range of health problems, since most health problems are allergy-based. If there were a book on a particular health problem, then they could help their friends to gain a better understanding of NAET®.

Because the NAET® approach to each particular health issue has some similar foundations, I must repeat certain information in each book. (It does not feel right to give partial information in one book and advise readers to buy other books to find the remaining information.) So, if someone would like to know about NAET® and skin disorders, they only have to buy this book. All pertinent information is given here. Of course, readers who would like to further educate themselves, or help other family or friends with different health issues, can buy other NAET® books.

Readers interested in learning more about acupuncture meridians and the possible pathological symptoms, or diagnostic testing and evaluations to detect allergies, should read my book "*Say Good-bye to Illness*". All of my NAET® books and other educational products are available at our Website: www.naet.com. Alternatively, readers who wish to further enhance their understanding may find additional publications of interest in the bibliography section of this book.

Stay allergy-free and enjoy better HEALTH!

Devi S. Nambudripad, M.D., D.C., L.Ac., Ph.D. (Acu.)

Introduction

*I*t is everyone's right to eat the foods they find available and enjoyable, and then digest, assimilate, and absorb the essential nutrients from these foods without any trouble. It is also everyone's right to be healthy and happy with the people and the environment in which they live. If people can accomplish this, they can say that they are in a healthy condition. If they are not able to do this, they need to see a NAET® Specialist.

People who do not have a personal experience with NAET® might be confused by that statement. However, people who do have personal experience with NAET® would agree, because NAET® can indeed help people achieve health and happiness.

People have been suffering from various skin disorders for hundreds of years, yet no one knows the cause of many of these skin disorders. Most health care practitioners identify and treat the disorders according to the patient's symptoms. Symptomatic treatments work very well most of the time, and when the symptoms are gone, the doctor and the patient are happy. Sometimes, when the symptomatic treatments may not work, the doctor is puzzled, and patients are confused and disappointed. This is a frequent scenario in today's world.

What Is NAET®?

NAET® is a noninvasive, drug-free, natural solution that eliminates allergy-related skin disorders using a blend of selective energy balancing, testing, and treatment procedures from Oriental medicine (acupuncture/acupressure), Western medicine, chiropractic, kinesiology, and nutritional disciplines of medicine. Most skin disorders are caused by allergy, whether we realize it or not.

According to NAET® theory, some "software problems" in the brain-computer (perhaps similar to a virus in the desktop computer) are the cause of allergies and allergy-related illnesses.

NAET® is a way to reprogram the brain to its original state. NAET® is the computer virus treatment that helps the brain remove the faulty programs and replace them with the correct programs.

NAET® also stresses the importance of lifestyle changes. Consuming non-allergic foods and drinks, living in a non-allergic environment, using non-allergic materials, associating with non-allergic people, exercising adequately, and maintaining sound mental health, can all be lifestyle changes. This could mean eating more nutritious meals, and eliminating emotional conflicts and unhappy situations.

NAET® is not a magic cure for anything. It is pure hard work based on Oriental medicine theory. If a person is not willing to work hard, NAET® is not for that person. If a person is willing to work hard and make lifestyle changes, that person can find relief from any allergy-based symptoms, including those mentioned in this and other books by this author (see the bibliography section under "Allergy Relief"). This author has treated every one of those allergy-based problems successfully with NAET®. However, if the patient's presenting problems are not due to allergies, then NAET® is not the way to treat that patient's problems.

The main application of NAET® is to remove the adverse reactions between the body and other substances. The result is that the body recovers its natural ability to absorb and assimilate essential nutrients, and its natural ability to eliminate unwanted toxicities.

When a person is treated with NAET® for known allergens, that person will no longer react: the items become non-allergic. When these items contact or enter the body, if the items are not useful to the body, the body will eliminate them naturally, without creating havoc in the immune system.

This book helps people understand how allergies affect them, and how allergies produce illnesses that mimic severe skin disorders. Some people require several NAET® treatment sessions, while others may require only a few sessions if they have only mild or hidden allergies. At some point in the treatment program, NAET® Specialists teach their patients self-testing procedures that can be done at home. By reading this book, patients can learn how allergies and allergy-related illness can now be controlled.

NAET® was developed by Dr. Devi S. Nambudripad, who has been treating patients with this technique since 1983, and teaching other health professionals since 1989. NAET® procedures have now been taught to more than 10,000 licensed healthcare professionals world-wide. For more information on NAET® or to find a NAET® Specialist in any region of the world, visit the NAET® Website at www.naet.com.

How Do People Know if They Have Allergies?

Anyone who experiences any unusual physical or emotional symptoms, without any obvious reason, can suspect an allergy.

Who Should Use This Book?

Anyone who is suffering from allergies or allergy-related skin disorders (eczema, itching, hives, rashes, acne, psoriasis, candidiasis, athlete's foot, hair loss, etc.) should read this book. This natural, noninvasive technique is ideal to treat infants, children, adults, and seniors who suffer from mild to severe allergic reactions, without altering their current plan of treatment. NAET® encourages the use of all medications, supplements, or other therapies prescribed by the patient's regular physician, while going through the NAET® program. When the patient's condition improves, that patient's regular physician can reduce or alter the dosage of drugs, or otherwise modify their treatment plan as needed.

How Is This Book Organized?

Chapter 1:   Describes **symptoms and causes** of eczema, acne, and other common skin disorders, and includes some stories of how people with these problems found freedom from their suffering

Chapter 2:   Explains **allergens that trigger skin disorders**, and includes stories of people whose skin disorders were caused by these allergens

Chapter 3:   Describes **diagnostic methods** (Western medicine, Oriental medicine, and NAET® approaches, including self-help) for determining which allergies are causing symptoms

Chapter 4:   Describes **treatment** (Western medicine, Oriental medicine, and NAET® approaches, including self-help) for eczema, acne, and other common skin disorders

Chapter 5:   Provides further insight through a collection of additional **NAET® success stories**

Glossary: Defines the medical terms used in this book (and often found in other materials on this topic)

Resources: Provides additional sources of education, products, and services for allergy-relief support

Bibliography: Offers ideas for further detailed reading on topics discussed in this book

Index: Helps readers find particular information of interest, quickly and easily

CHAPTER 1

WHAT ARE COMMON SKIN DISORDERS?

Understanding Symptoms and Causes

OVERVIEW

Freedom From Eczema:
Mr. Villanueva's Journey

*E*czema can have excruciating effects. Attorney Carlito S. Villanueva, F.P.M. shared this story about the heavy toll it took on his life in the Philippines, and how his NAET® Specialist, Milagros Ting, B.S.N., B.S. Pharmacy, helped him on his journey to freedom.

I consider myself generally a healthy person.I have not suffered anything more serious than common colds, flu, rhinitis allergy, and occasional allergic reactions to some foods and drugs.

That was until the year 2004 and at an age above 50. During the later part of that year, I started to be bothered by some itchiness on my back, initially in a small area, until I felt it was spreading to a bigger portion of my back.

With days passing by, and itchiness increasing in intensity, I decided to consult a dermatologist at the nearby United Doctors Hospital. The finding was comforting. The doctor found nothing more serious than acne and accordingly prescribed some ointment and soap that I should be using. I thought that was the end of my problem.

But I was wrong.

My condition did not improve. The rashes that originated in my back were gradually spreading to my upper torso and started to manifest even on my face. I decided to see another dermatologist. A friend mentioned the name of a lady dermatologist holding clinic in front of San Lazaro Hospital. My friend told me this lady doctor has a superb reputation as a dermatologist. Feeling a fresh ray hope, I did not wait for another day to see her. In her clinic, she meticulously examined my bare body and the unsightly rashes that pestered me. Specimen tissue was taken off my arm for skin biopsy. The next meeting I had with her, she showed me the result of the biopsy. The findings were couched in some technical term, but the end sentence of the report that I understood spelled it out: I WAS SUFFERING FROM A CERTAIN CONDITION CONSISTENT WITH ECZEMA!

What followed was an every-other-day visit to my lady dermatologist, for two weeks. There was a time when this doctor was injecting each of the rashes in my body with something I could only surmise as a steroid. Despite all these treatments and procedures, I did not feel any improvement in my condition. My feeling was… it was even getting worse.

And I stopped seeing the doctor.

Frustrated and not knowing what to do, I had to give way to the advice of some old people that my condition was not within the competence of modern medicine to cure. They said I got the ire of some powerful but unfriendly fairy or dwarfs and the only remedy

I could resort to was to seek the help of a faith healer who has the power to free me from the spell of this fairy or dwarf.

And so, the start of some of the most ridiculous experiences I ever had in my life began. I consulted no less than four of these faith healers. I was forced by necessity to travel hundred of kilometers away from the city to see them. Each one of them had a different finding, theory, or diagnosis of what was ailing me. One of them said I was under the power of a witch who was commissioned by somebody to harm me. Still another one said I accidentally stepped on an ant hill that served as a dwelling place of a fairy while playing golf, or probably I peed on this ant hill.

I had to join these faith healers in certain rituals that they performed to drive the supposedly mysterious power that possessed me. We had to offer foods to certain unseen elements; prayed to certain gods other than the God I know; joined them in their weird encantation. At one treatment session, I had to suffer the pain of fire from a lighted candle, as this candle was trained on the various part of my body where I had rashes. Not the least of all, I had to endure the horrendous taste of some concoctions I was asked to drink, and experience bathing in water full of all sort of leaves and wild flowers.

In the end nothing positive happened. In fact my condition was growing worse as my frustration became more intense. After some soul searching, once again, I decided to go back to the fold of modern medicine. I sought confinement at the Manila Doctors Hospital where I was attended by a friend and former work associate who was the top allergist in that Hospital. Several laboratory tests were done on me but none of the results could point out conclusively what was really ailing me. Since Christmas was approaching, I decided to leave the hospital after a week of confinement as I did not want to spend Christmas in the hospital.

It was a sad Christmas for me. My health was failing with rashes now practically covering my entire body and face. I was a

*complete picture of gloom as my physical appearance was slowly
turning into nothing more than the shadow of my former self. I spent
time mostly inside my room trying to keep my sanity intact. I did not
want to be seen by anybody as I grew tired answering the question
"WHAT HAPPENED TO YOU?" from friends and relatives.*

*Then again, upon the urging of a client who swore a derma-
tologist she knew at Makati Medical Center can cure my ailment, I
went to that hospital full of new hope. Upon seeing me, the woman
dermatologist made a quick decision: I had to be confined in the
hospital. And so it happened over the objection of my wife.*

*I spent thirteen (13) agonizing days in that hospital. Everyday
my hope was dwindling, slowly ebbing like the setting sun in the
late afternoon. Every morning, I saw the blank and puzzled face of
my dermatologist who nonetheless would try to impress a horde of
her students who accompanied her as she lectured on the various
theories and probabilities of what was causing my ailment. I was
the guinea pig. Here I was given various intravenous treatments
and taking daily no less than sixteen (16) varieties of very expensive drugs. If you have heard of a shotgun-approach to treatment I
thought this was it! My dermatologist did not seem to consider that
some of those drugs may have been causing some adverse effect on
me, like difficulty in breathing. And every time I would complain
about it, my attending nurse was quick in administering a nebulizer,
the taste of which I cursed every minute that it was in my mouth.*

*My condition, instead of improving, got worse in this hospital.
I ballooned from my usual weight of 155lbs to 187lbs probably
because of an overdose of steroid. My entire body was wrapped
by bandages like a mummy every evening to cover the steroid ointment applied all over my entire body. I felt at that time that if I had
stayed a few more days in this hospital, death would be a certainty.
I asked to be discharged, and as I left the hospital, I noticed that
what used to be a single name of my dermatologist posted at the
door of my hospital room increased to seven (7). It then dawned*

on me that for every little complaint I mentioned to my dermatologist, she referred me to another specialist in the hospital.

Finally home again, my wife who had been patiently looking and taking care of me day and night thought that I should try her idea this time – that of seeing an herbalist or a practicing health naturalist. Desperate but always ready to try anything, I agreed to throw what I consider was my last card.

This health practitioner, a young and beautiful lady, holds a doctorate in Chemistry from the University of the Philippines. She was thus addressed as "doctor" and I suspect many of her patients thought she was a doctor of medicine. Her clinic in Ortigas Avenue was always full of patients, many of whom would readily swear that many impossible cases, ranging from the dreadful cancer to the terrifying Alzheimer's diseases, found cure in her.

Seeing my condition for the first time, she gave herself a deadline of four months within which to deliver me from my ailment. The long process of taking very expensive herbal medicine started. In a short time, she succeeded in putting back my former weight. The various laboratory tests done on me after some period of treatment also showed that all my internal organs were back in their normal condition. After four months though, and beyond, there was little improvement in my skin condition. She had given me all of the herbal medicine available, and I had spent a fortune for them, yet my skin condition showed very little improvement.

I was resigned to my hideous appearance when I was next seen by a doctor of medicine (a referral of a court mediator) who was a fellow of Biological Medicine and also a fellow of the International Board of Chelation Therapy. After seeing me a few times and after evaluating the result of a lab test that was even processed abroad (which noted nothing more than an elevated mercury level in my blood), she seemed to have readily given up my case. Instead of pursuing a treatment, she referred me to a lady named *MILAGROS TING, a kind and amiable lady who is a practitioner of a system of treatment or method called Nambudripad's Allergy Elimination Technique (NAET®). I came to know later that the doctor who referred me to Ms. Ting had a son who was suffering from a severe case of asthma. He was cured by Ms. Ting using the NAET® system. I also realized that in Ms. Ting's clinic I was in the company of no ordinary people and personalities who were all seeking treatment from her. She must be good, I thought.*

Ms. Ting drew a program that I would be undergoing for a certain period of time under the NAET® system. But after observing and feeling the application of treatment done on me, there was a serious doubt that almost instantly gripped me. I felt I was forcing myself to believe something that I found not only funny but ridiculous – I mean the system! Part of the treatment process involved several test tubes of various kind and sizes, the contents of which I had not even a vague idea. While lying flat on my stomach and holding one or two of these test tubes, Ms. Ting would run on my back a gadget that operates and sounds like a staccato massager. After the treatment session that lasted 10 to 15 minutes, I was to diet or avoid certain food or drink for 24 hours. The process was both too simplistic and highly unorthodox. As a lawyer trained to think like a lawyer, pursuing the treatment became a taunting dilemma for me.

How could I expect cure from this nonsensical and bizarre system of treatment? I could not help but ask myself.

But then, my doubt slowly turned into faith when, on my second visit to Ms. Ting (three days after my first treatment session with her), she noticed what I myself noticed: The redness and bloated appearance of my face was now less pronounced. For the first time, I felt my ebbing hope about my skin condition suddenly rekindled. Gradually, I saw the improvement of my condition after every visit I made to Ms. Ting. I was in her clinic initially twice a week until the frequency was reduced to once a week, then later, at my option, when I wanted to come. It is now close to one year that I have been undergoing treatment with her, and my condition, except for some slight discoloration on my face and arms, is almost back to normal. Ms. Ting is saying that, of similar cases she had treated before, it takes one to two years before a person of my same predicament could be completely cured and cleansed.

Who cares if it is two years if I could see again my bygone self? Thank God there is NAET® and a kind and amiable Ms. Milagros Ting who practices it in the Philippines.

(Figures 1-1 and 1-2 on the next page show Mr. Villanueva before and after NAET® treatment.)

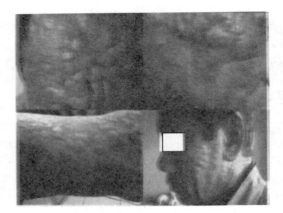

Figure 1-1. Severe eczema before NAET®.

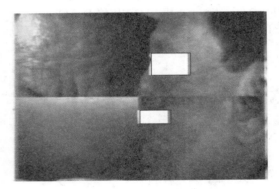

Figure 1-2. Severe eczema after NAET®.

History of Skin Disorders

Skin and skin disorders have interested medical practitioners from all disciplines since the earliest days of civilization.

Early Descriptions of Skin Problems

Many centuries ago different terms were used to describe skin conditions. Hippocrates in Greece, Celsus in Italy, and others in the Middle East made early contributions to dermatology (study of the skin) by compounding materials to combat the common skin disorders of that time: alopecia (hair loss), pediculosis (lice infestation), scabies (mite infestation), pruritis (intense itching), and leprosy (infectious disease of the skin, peripheral nerves, and mucous membranes). The first clinical descriptions of skin conditions and their treatments date back to 1600 BC in ancient Egypt, where medicinal healers treated such conditions as psoriasis, ulcers, alopecia, and scabies. Hippocrates, Pluto, and Aristotle (all ancient Greek physicians) adopted Egyptian healing traditions for skin disorders, and coined many of the technical terms, such as alopecia, exanthem (rash), lichen (a fungus), psoriasis, leprosy, gangrene (death of body tissue), and edema (swelling), that we still use in dermatology today. The word "derma" was coined by Hippocrates, the Father of Medicine, and has been used ever since. The first English book on cutaneous disorders, *De Morbis Cutaneis*, was written by the English surgeon Daniel Turner and published in 1714. For the first time, Turner attempted to classify skin conditions according to body area. In 1790, Robert Willan, a general practitioner in London, expanded classification of skin diseases in his book, *Description and Treatment of Cutaneous Diseases*, and introduced new clinical entities such as erythema nodosum (inflammatory reaction deep in the skin). He was awarded a gold medal by the Medical Society of London and is considered the Father of modern dermatology in the Western world.

Development of a Medical Specialty

Toward the end of the 19th century, the practice of dermatology emerged, as doctors – known as dermatologists – began specializing in the skin and its disorders. Since then, the study and practice of dermatology as a field of its own has continued to grow. During the late 1930s and early 1940s important treatment advancements were made. It is interesting to observe that as time progressed, scientific advancements included cures and eradication of certain skin disorders such as leprosy, as well as entirely new sets of disorders such as dermatitis from chemical exposures. (As civilization moved from an agricultural to industrial age, chemical exposures were more common, and this form of dermatitis was more severe than the plant-contact dermatitis that had first been described nearly 2000 years ago by Pliny the Younger as "a severe itching from cutting pine trees".) Treatment and experimentation in dermatology has progressed significantly, as topical emollients, steroids, and antibiotics developed for use in combating inflammation and providing symptomatic relief (even though the true cause of many skin disorders remained a mystery).

Current Pressing Problems, and Hope

Skin disorders — especially eczema and acne — are still abundant, active, aggressive, and increasing in frequency, yet many still do not know of the actual cause or proper cure of these disorders. Fortunately, there is hope. According to NAET® theory, allergies cause 99% of skin disorders, and these skin disorders can be eliminated with NAET® allergy desensitization treatment.

What Is an Allergy?

An allergy is a condition whereby one person has unusual sensitivity to one or more substances that may be harmless or even beneficial to the majority of other people. The literal meaning of allergy comes from the Greek word "allos", which translates to "altered action" or "reaction". The term allergy was first proposed in 1906 by an Austrian pediatrician, Clemens Von Pirquet (1874-1929), who worked with tuberculosis patients, studying the immune system and its connection with what we now call allergic reactions. It was Pirquet who developed a scratch test for tuberculosis, a forerunner of the allergy scratch testing done in many clinics today. By combining the two Greek words "allos" (altered) and "ergion" (action or reactivity), Pirquet created the word allergy, literally meaning "altered reactivity". This describes a person's biological hypersensitivity to substances, which in similar amounts and circumstances, are harmless to most people.

Somewhere around mid 400 BC, nearly 2500 years ago, Hippocrates noted that cheese caused severe reactions in some men, while others could eat and enjoy it with no unpleasant after effects. Three hundred years later, the Roman philosopher Lucretius said, "what is food for some may be fierce poison for others". This was the original source of the expression, "one man's meat is another man's poison".

The activation of immunoglobulin type E (IgE) antibodies causes what Western medical professionals call "true" allergies. However, millions of people experience various allergic symptoms every day in varying degrees without producing these antibodies; such reactions can be called intolerance or hypersensitivity.

When the body is exposed to what it thinks is a foreign and dangerous substance, a normal immune system will immediately release chemical mediators (antibodies) appropriate to the condition to defend the body. Within a few seconds, the body comes to a settlement with the foreign substance, without causing any obvious symptoms of illness. But when the immune system perceives what should be harmless as a dangerous intruder, and then stimulates production of antibodies to defend the body, the body does not come to a settlement with the allergen. Instead, this first contact initiates the baby step of an allergic reaction inside the body, producing a few antibodies and storing them in reserve for future use.

In most people, a first contact or initial sensitization will usually not produce many symptoms. During the second exposure to the allergen, the body will alert the previously produced antibodies to action, producing more noticeable symptoms (particularly in someone with a weaker immune system). But often, with the third exposure, the threatened immune system will begin serious action by producing massive amounts of antibodies to defend against the invader, causing some kind of allergic reaction. The areas of the body most commonly affected by allergic reactions are the skin, eyes, nose, throat, mouth, rectum, and vaginal mucosa. In sensitive individuals, contact with allergens can produce eczema and other common skin disorders in varying degrees, from mild itching in one area to severe symptoms covering the whole body.

A List of Common Skin Disorders

Skin disorders can generally be described according to:

- **Location** on the body where the condition appears
- **Appearance** of the skin
- **Contributing factor** (manifestation)

The most common locations on the body where skin disorders appear include the hands, feet, groin, scalp, and face.

The most common appearances of skin disorders include some form of rash, inflammation, pimples, pus-filled bumps, blisters, dry scales, hardening, hair loss, itching, and/or pain.

The most common contributing factors include infections, pigmentation disorders, gravitational force, infestations/bites, and skin tumors.

Because there are so many kinds of skin disorders, it can help to better understand them in categories. Although many skin disorders could be categorized in more than one way (location, appearance, or contributing factor), this simplified list categorizes disorders by either general appearance or contributing factor. Some of the more common disorders — eczema, acne, psoriasis, candidiasis, athlete's foot, and hair loss — are described in more detail in this chapter.

Skin Disorders Grouped by Appearance

Eczema & other disorders with persistent or recurring skin rashes, such as:

Acne & other disorders with pimples or pus-containing tender bumps, such as:

- Atopic dermatitis
- Chronic dermatitis
- Contact dermatitis
- Dermatitis
- Diaper rash
- Discoid eczema
- Dishyidrotic eczema
- Foot eczema
- Groin eczema
- Hand eczema
- Lichen simplex chronicus
- Miliaria (heat rash)
- Nummular dermatitis
- Perioral dermatitis
- Seborrhoeic eczema (cradle cap)
- Urticaria (hives)
- Xerotic eczema

- Acne conglobata
- Acne cosmetica
- Acne due to weather changes
- Acne excoriee
- Acne fulminans
- Acne keloidalis nuchae
- Acne medicamentosa
- Acne rosacea
- Acne vulgaris
- Baby acne and milia
- Chloracne
- Cystic acne
- Folliculitis
- Hidradenitis suppurativa
- Keratosis pilaris
- Occupational acne
- Pyoderma faciale

Psoriasis & other disorders with scales or elevation of skin without pus, such as:

- Erythroderma
- Grover's disease
- Ichthyosis
- Lichen planus
- Pityriasis rosea
- Pityriasis rubra pilaris
- Seborrheic dermatitis (dandruff)

Baldness and Hair Loss:

- Alopecia areata
- Alopecia totalis
- Alopecia universalis

Vessicular disorders with blisters but not rash or itching, such as:

- Bed sores
- Bullous pemphigoid
- Dermatitis herpetiformis
- Friction blisters
- Gestational phemigoid
- Pemphigus

Skin hardening:

- Scleroderma

Pigmentation disorders:

- Moles
- Photosensitivity
- Porphyria
- Melasma
- Vitiligo

Skin Disorders Grouped by Contributing Factors

Infection:

Fungal infections:
- **Candidiasis**
- Ringworm (tinea)
- Tinea barbae (beard)
- Tinea capitis (scalp)
- Tinea corporis (body)
- Tinea cruris (groin: jock itch)
- Tinea oncomycosis (nails)
- **Tinea pedis (athlete's foot)**
- Tinea unguium
- Tinea versicolor

Bacterial infections:
- Impetigo
- Cellulitis
- Erysipelas

Viral infections:
- Warts
- Molluscum contagiosum
- Herpes simplex (cold sores)
- Herpes zoster (shingles)

Gravitational force:

- Spider veins
- Stasis dermatitis

Infestation or bite:

- Scabies
- Lice infection
- Tick bite
- Hookworms (creeping eruption)
- Fleas (tungiasis)

Skin tumors:

Benign skin tumors:
- Skin tags
- Dermatofibroma
- Keloid
- Keratoacanthoma
- Sebaceous cyst

Skin cancer:
- Actinic keratosis
- Basal cell carcinoma
- Bowen's Disease
- Kaposi's sarcoma
- Malignant melanoma

Note: Most skin disorders including eczema are a direct result of some kind of allergies, or are somehow allergy-based. In this book, only allergy-based skin conditions are discussed. Patients who suspect that their skin disorder is caused by anything else should consult a qualified medical professional who can help find a solution.

ECZEMA

The word eczema comes from Greek and means 'to boil over'. The medical terms eczema and dermatitis are often used interchangably, and describe many different skin conditions. Like many allergic conditions, the severity of the disease can vary, and in some cases it can look very unpleasant. However, eczema is not contagious.

What Are the Symptoms of Eczema?

Eczema is generally an inflammation of the dermis and epidermis (upper layers of the skin) on any part of the body. Symptoms include a range of persistent or recurring skin rashes characterized by redness, swelling, itching, dryness, crusting, flaking, blistering, cracking, oozing, and/or bleeding. In general, in the xerotic form of eczema the skin is dry, itchy, and cracked; whereas in the discoid form of eczema there are distinct round spots that are dry or oozing. Any of these conditions can also cause varying degrees of pain.

What Causes Eczema?

The exact cause of eczema is not known. Genetic predisposition may be a contributing factor. Other conditions that may contribute include:

- Allergies
- Gravitational force
- Hormonal changes
- Scratching
- Injury
- Underlying (totally unrelated) health disorder

According to NAET® theory, one of the major causes for all types of eczema may be an allergy to something one is eating, drinking, or touching, at home, outdoors, or at work. Areas of work with a high risk include: hairdressing, nursing, house cleaning, cooking, engineering, writing, typing, working with computers, animal grooming, wood carving, plastering, roofing, and installing ceramic tile, marble floor, concrete, or carpet, as well as various kinds of carpentry. Chapter 2 describes allergies in more detail.

How Common Is Eczema?

Eczema is seen among people of all ages, in every city, and in every country.

In the United States, statistics from the National Institute of Allergy and Infectious Diseases and the National Institute of Arthritis and Musculoskeletal and Skin Diseases showed that:

- More than 15 million people have symptoms of atopic dermatitis (one common form of eczema).
- Eczema cases account for 10-20% of all visits to dermatologists.
- 65% of patients develop eczema symptoms before they are one year old, and 90% develop these eczema skin symptoms before they are five years old.

The Australian Bureau of Statistics' National Health Survey indicated that:

- Over 221,200 people, over half of whom were women, self-reported having dermatitis and eczema in 2005.

In England, the Department of Health 2005-2006 Hospital Episode Statistics showed that:

- More than 10,700 hospital episodes were for dermatitis and eczema; 51% of these episodes were for women, and 49% were for men.
- Over 90% of hospital consultations for dermatitis and eczema required hospital admission.

Other interesting statistics include the following:

- Atopic (allergic) dermatitis is the most common skin condition in children younger than 11 years old; the percentage of children diagnosed with this condition has increased from 3% in the 1960s to 10% in the 1990s.
- Acute urticaria (hives) is common, affecting up to 20% of the population at some time in their lives; half of those affected continue to have symptoms for more than six months.
- Contact dermatitis and other forms of eczema were diagnosed in over 8.5 million physician office visits and in 499,000 hospital outpatient visits.
- Atopic dermatitis is one of the most common skin diseases, particularly in infants and children; approximately 9% of the United States population is affected by atopic dermatitis, and this number appears to be increasing.

What Are the Complications of Eczema?

Eczema and related conditions can have significant psychological effects among both caretakers and sufferers of eczema. Among caretakers of children with eczema:

- Stress takes a real toll: 52% feel they have no control over their child's condition 23% never get a good night's sleep, and 5% feel the whole household is disrupted.

Among people with eczema:

- Relationships suffer: 29% feel people do not want to touch them, 21% have had difficulty forming a relationship, and 21% cannot bear to have anyone touch them.
- Self-image issues arise: 73% of sufferers worry about their appearance, 63% of sufferers do not want others to see their skin, 47% cannot wear the clothes that they want to wear, 40% avoid cosmetics when in flare, 31% avoid wearing shorts/skirts/t-shirts when in flare, and 27% hate seeing themselves in the mirror.
- Self-esteem issues arise: 47% are embarrassed when they are with people whom they do not know very well, 27% have been teased or bullied because of their eczema, 26% worry about meeting people, 20% worry that people will not accept them, 17% have no self confidence, and 11% want to stay away from others altogether.

Eczema affects many people — one in five children and one in twelve adults — and when one person in a family has eczema, everyone in that family can be affected. The person with eczema often can do nothing to stop themselves from scratching, and has to live everyday with painful, cracked and often bleeding skin. That person's parents, guardians, or caregivers can be left feeling helpless, guilty, and exhausted through lack of sleep and worry. Children with eczema may awaken several times at night because they have scratched so much they need change of clothes, bed linen, and need more skin moisturizers or creams to apply to soothe the skin. This can take its toll on parents and other family members who need enough sleep to perform daily activities. Caring for the sick child takes a lot of effort. Siblings can also feel left out because their parents may be spending most of their time with the sick child and leaving the healthy child unattended. The financial strain associated with good medical care may also create significant tension among parents and other family members. Siblings may become angry and frustrated if they are forced to sacrifice money and other possessions towards the health care cost of the sick child. Clearly, many factors can contribute to an ongoing tension in all family members.

ACNE

What Are the Symptoms of Acne?

Acne generally refers to pimples or pus-containing lesions commonly found on the face, neck, or upper body. There are many different types of acne (see details later in this section). In some people, symptoms may disappear after a few days. However in other people, symptoms can persist for a long time, and when symptoms eventually do disappear, deep scars can remain, both physically and emotionally.

What Causes Acne?

In general, acne occurs when bacteria-filled hair follicles become inflamed. Often, this is from the effects of hormones on the sebaceous glands (which are glands in the skin that secrete oil, or sebum, into hair follicles). For example, androgens (male sex hormones) stimulate sebaceous gland secretion into dilated hair follicles that contain bacteria. The bacteria, usually *Propionibacterium acnes* and *Staphylococcus epidermidis* (which are normal skin flora), secrete lipase (an enzyme). This enzyme interacts with sebum to produce free fatty acids, which provoke inflammation. Also, the hair follicles produce more keratin (a tough hair-forming protein), which joins with the sebum to form a plug in the dilated follicle. However, the exact *cause* of this process is not known. Several factors that may be linked to triggering acne include:

- Genetic factors (family history)
- Stress, through increased output of hormones from the adrenal (stress) glands

- Hyperactive sebaceous glands, secondary to the hyper-activity of hormones (female hormones, male hormones, adrenal hormones, birth control pills; many females experience an acne flare-up during their first few menstrual cycles after starting or discontinuing hormonal contraceptives)
- Accumulation of dead skin cells (not cleaning the skin enough or properly, or allergy to the skin itself)
- Bacteria in the pores, to which the body becomes 'allergic'
- Prior bacterial infection
- Skin irritation (from trauma, rubbing, or tight clothing, or scratching of any sort)
- Cosmetics with ingredients to which the body is allergic
- Any medication containing halogens (iodides, chlorides, bromides), corticosteroids, lithium, barbiturates, or androgens
- Exposure to high levels of chlorine compounds, particularly chlorinated dioxins
- Extreme weather conditions (heat, cold, humidity)
- Various foods, especially, greasy and fried foods
- Food allergies that trigger acne in individuals who have intolerances and hypersensitivities include: carbonated drinks, coffee, partially skimmed milk, instant breakfast drink, sherbet, cottage cheese, cream cheese, milk ingredients (casein, albumin), seafood (an allergy to iodine), refined sugars, processed food with high carbohydrates, soft drinks, white bread, bleached bread, food high in fat and sugar, chocolate, potato chips, spices, French fries, deep fried foods, deep fried mozzarella sticks, deep fried food that contains fats and sugar (for example: donuts, dumplings), spicy foods, hot pepper sauce, superheated oils, vinegars, certain sea salts, corn chips, tomato sauce, genetically modified foods, food additives, food colorings, gelatin, gums, soft drinks, highly acidic or basic foods, and vitamin and mineral supplements, vitamin C, and tropical fruits like mango and star fruits

How Common Is Acne?

Acne is a common skin disorder often seen among teenagers. Three out of four teenagers have acne, probably due to increased hormone activity, poor dietary habits (drinking carbonated sodas, coffee, eating chocolates, refined sugar products, and deep fried foods such as donuts and mozzarella sticks), poor cleansing habits, and lots of allergies. Most adolescents and adults have acne at some time in their life. Statistics show that nearly 17 million people in the United States have some form of acne, making it the most common skin disorder in this country.

What Are the Different Types of Acne?

Some of the more common forms of acne can be grouped according to their general symptoms (location and appearance), or according to specific causes. The types of acne best described by specific location and appearance include:

- Acne vulgaris
- Acne rosacea
- Acne keloidalis nuchae
- Acne conglobata
- Acne fulminans
- Pyoderma faciale
- Milia (baby acne)

The types of acne that are best described by specific causes (and are in fact named accordingly) include:

- Acne cosmetica (caused by cosmetics)
- Acne excoriee (caused by habitual picking)
- Occupational acne (usually a result of contact with mineral oil or petroleum)
- Chloracne (exposure to chlorine compounds)

- Acne medicamentosa (response to certain medications)
- Acne due to weather change

Another form of acne with various subtypes and causes is:

- Folliculitis

Types of Acne Best Described by Location and Appearance

Acne Vulgaris

- **Location.** Painful bumps — commonly referred to as pimples, spots, or zits — usually occur on the face, chest, back, shoulders and upper arms.
- **Appearance (typical).** Typical acne lesions include comedones (whiteheads and blackheads), papules (bumps), and pustules (pus-filled bumps):
  - o Comedones can appear as small white spots (whiteheads) or black spots (blackheads); whiteheads usually resolve fairly quickly, while blackheads can often take a long time to clear.
  - o Papules are inflamed, red, tender bumps with no head.
  - o Pustules (common zits) are similar to whiteheads, but are inflamed and appear as red circles with a white or yellow center.
- **Appearance (severe).** Severe acne vulgaris involves nodules or cysts, which are more painful, inflamed, pus-filled, or reddish bumps that can easily lead to scarring or serious infections.
  - o Nodules are large, hard bumps under the skin's surface
  - o Cysts (cystic acne) can appear similar to a nodule, but are pus-filled and at least 5mm in diameter.
  - o **Notes:** (1) One should never attempt to squeeze a nodule or cyst lesion. This may cause severe trauma to the skin, causing a deeper infection and more

painful inflammation, resulting in the lesion lasting for months longer than it normally would. It is very important for a person with nodules or cysts to see a dermatologist. (2) Cystic acne usually occurs in males, generally persists beyond the age of 20 years, and may lead to permanent scarring.

- **Cause.** Acne vulgaris begins with a blockage in the hair follicle, followed by hyperkeratinization (excessive development of the tough protein in the outer layer of skin) and formation of a plug of keratin (the tough protein) and sebum (oily secretion from the sebaceous glands near follicles). Enlargement of sebaceous glands and an increase in sebum production occur with increased androgen production. Bacterial overgrowth of *Propionibacterium acnes* can cause inflammation. In response to the bacterial and yeast populations, the skin inflames, producing visible bumps.
  - o **Whiteheads:** Whiteheads result when a pore is completely blocked, trapping sebum, bacteria, and dead skin cells, causing a white appearance on the surface. Whiteheads normally clear fairly quickly.
  - o **Blackheads:** Blackheads result when a pore is only partially blocked, allowing some of the trapped sebum, bacteria, and dead skin cells to slowly drain to the surface. The black color is not caused by dirt. Rather, it is a reaction of the skin's own pigment, melanin, reacting with the oxygen in the air. Blackheads can often take a long time to clear.
- **How common is it?** Acne vulgaris is the most common form of acne, usually developing around puberty (often between ages 15 and 18), although it can appear as early as age 8. Although acne strikes boys more often and more severely than girls, it usually occurs in girls at an earlier age and tends to last longer, sometimes into adulthood.

- **Complications.** After resolution of severe acne, scars may remain. In addition, because acne vulgaris usually appears during adolescence when people already tend to be socially insecure, the main effects of acne vulgaris are psychological, such as low self-esteem and low self-worth, inferiority complex, depression, or suicide.

Acne Rosacea

- **Location.** Rosacea normally affects the central face and across the cheeks, nose, or forehead; less commonly, rosacea can affect the neck and chest.

- **Appearance.** Rosacea begins as erythema (flushing and redness) often from exercise, changes in temperature, and cleansing; it appears as a red rash, which is often accompanied by bumps, pimples, and skin blemishes. Rosacea progresses into one or more of the four identified rosacea subtypes:

  o **Erythematotelangiectatic rosacea,** which is marked by permanent redness (erythema) with a tendency to flush and blush easily. It is also common to have small blood vessels visible near the surface of the skin and possibly burning or itching sensations.

  o **Papulopustular rosacea,** which is marked by some permanent redness with red bumps (papules) and some pus filled (pustules).

  o **Phymatous rosacea,** which is marked by thickening skin, irregular surface nodularities, and enlargement. Phymatous rosacea can affect the nose (rhinophyma), chin (gnatophyma), forehead (metophyma), cheeks, eyelids (blepharophyma), and ears (otophyma). Small blood vessels visible near the surface of the skin (telangiectasias) may be present.

  o **Ocular rosacea,** which is marked by red, dry and irritated eyes and eyelids. Some other symptoms include foreign body sensations, itching and burning.

- ○ **Note:** Rosacea can be confused with acne vulgaris and/ or seborrheic dermatitis. Since rosacea is primarily a facial diagnosis, the presence of rash on the scalp or ears suggests a different or coexisting diagnosis.
- **Cause.** The first signs of rosacea are said to be persistent redness due to exercise, changes in temperature, and cleansing. Most experts believe that rosacea is a disorder where the blood vessels become damaged when repeatedly dilated by stimuli. The damage causes the vessels to dilate too easily and stay dilated for longer periods of time or remain permanently dilated, resulting in flushing and redness. Triggers that cause episodes of flushing and blushing play a part in the development of rosacea. Triggers that can cause the face to become flushed inlcude exposure to extreme temperatures, strenuous exercise, heat from sunlight, severe sunburn, stress, anxiety, cold wind, and moving to a warm or hot environment from a cold one (such as going outside during the winter after being in a heated shop or office). Some foods and drinks that can trigger flushing include alcohol, foods and drinks containing caffeine (especially, hot tea and coffee), spicy food, and sugary food. Rosacea also has a genetic component: it affects fair-skinned people of mostly north-western European descent, and has been nicknamed by some in Ireland as the "curse of the Celts".
- **How common is it?** Acne rosacea is a common condition: statistics estimate that it affects over 45 million people worldwide, and approximately 13 million people in the United States. Women are more commonly affected; when men develop rosacea, the condition tends to be more severe. People of all ages can develop rosacea, but it is most common in the 30-50 age group.
- **Complications.** Rosacea sufferers often report periods of depression stemming from cosmetic disfigurement, painful burning sensations, and decreases in quality of life.

Acne Keloidalis Nuchae
(AKN, Pseudofolliculitis nuchae, Folliculitis keloidalis)
- **Location.** Acne keloidalis nuchae affects the nape of the neck.
- **Appearance.** Ingrown hairs become inflamed and lead to overgrown scar tissue that is called a hypertrophic scar, or keloid.
- **Cause.** This condition occurs when hairs on the back of the head and neck grow into the skin and become inflamed. These ingrown hairs usually occur following a short haircut on the back of the head and nape of the neck.
- **How common is it?** Acne keloidalis nuchae is an unusual skin condition, but is more common in people with stiff or curly hair on the neck, and in those with darker skin.

Acne Conglobata
- **Location.** Acne conglobata is found on the face, chest, back, groin, buttocks, armpits, thighs; in women, it can also be found under the breasts.
- **Appearance.** It is characterized by many large lesions, which are sometimes interconnected, along with widespread blackheads. Deep ulcers may form under the nodules, producing severe damage to the skin. Crusts may form over deeply ulcerated nodules; heavy irregular, disfiguring scarring and keloid-type scars result in most cases.
- **Note.** This is the most severe form of acne vulgaris and is more common in males. The age of onset for acne conglobata is usually between 18 and 30 years, and the condition can stay active for many years.
- **Cause.** The specific cause of this form of acne is not known.

Acne Fulminans (Acne Maligna)

- **Location.** Acne fulminans lesions occur on the face, torso and arms. This disorder may also cause symptoms in the joints and in the blood.
- **Appearance.** Lesions are papulopustular (small round bumps filled with pus), highly inflamed, and tender; they may eventually become ulcerative (open sores). Lesions are acute (onset is sudden), and accompanied by fever, weight loss and infammatory aching in the joints.
- **Note.** The sudden flare of acne fulminans can occur after unsuccessful treatment for another form of acne (acne conglobata).
- **Cause.** Acne fulminans is thought to be an immunologically induced disease. An elevated level of testosterone causes a rise in sebum and *Propionibacterium acnes* bacteria. The condition is commonly treated with steroids.

Pyoderma Faciale (Rosacea Fulminans)

- **Location.** Lesions appear on the cheeks, chin, and/or forehead.
- **Appearance.** The painful, large, red nodules (bumps), pustules (pus-filled blisters), and sores on the red areas in this unusual skin condition can resemble severe acne or rosacea, and likewise have the potential for later scarring.
- **Note.** Pyoderma faciale is seen in women 20-40 years old (males are not affected); onset is sudden, and may occur on the skin of a woman who has never had acne before. It usually does not last longer than one year.
- **Cause.** The specific cause of this form of acne is not known.

Baby Acne and Milia

- **Location.** Milia is seen on a baby's nose, chin, cheeks, and sometimes on the gums or roof of the mouth. Baby acne is seen only on the baby's forehead or cheeks.

- **Appearance.** Milia looks like pearly white bumps. Baby acne is more pronounced, with small red or white bumps, and may look worse when the baby is fussy or crying.
- **Note.** Many babies are born with milia. Baby acne often develops within the first three to four weeks after birth. Many babies have both conditions at the same time.
- **Cause.** Milia occur when tiny skin flakes become trapped in small pockets near the surface of the baby's skin. Baby acne is related to hormonal changes that stimulate oil glands in the skin. Milia affect boys and girls equally, but baby acne is more common in boys. Rarely, baby acne is a sign of a hormonal problem.

Types of Acne Best Described by Cause

Acne Cosmetica

Acne cosmetica is a term referring to acne caused by cosmetics. The prolonged use of cosmetics, especially those containing isopropyl myristate and greasy ingredients such as lanolin, can be responsible for this type of acne. The mechanism is presumably a chemically-induced plugging of the opening of the pilosebaceous gland (skin pore). Various cleansing creams, foundations, blushers, and moisturizers may contain chemicals that can aggravate acne. People may not attribute their reactions to their cosmetics at first, but may notice worsening symptoms after using certain face makeup, sunblock, or lip products.

Acne Medicamentosa

Acne medicamentosa is a response to certain medications. Adult females are highly prone to experience acne medicamentosa when they begin or stop taking birth control pills. One can also develop this disorder from reactions to other medications. Because acne is generally a disorder of the pilosebaceous glands, and is caused by hormones, it is hormone medication that most frequently triggers acne medicamentosa.

Occupational Acne

This is a type of acne that usually forms as the result of contact with mineral oil or petroleum. Occupational acne is a common condition suffered by motor mechanics who are frequently exposed to oils and grease.

Chloracne

Chloracne is an acne-like eruption of blackheads, cysts, and pustules (pus-filled bumps) associated with over-exposure to high levels of chlorine compounds, particularly certain halogenated aromatic hydrocarbons such as chlorinated dioxins and dibenzofurans.

Chloracne normally results from direct skin contact with chloracnegens — byproducts of many chemical processes, including the manufacture of herbicides such as Agent Orange and polychlorinated biphenyls (PCBs) — although ingestion and inhalation are also possible causative routes. PCB mixtures have been used for a variety of applications, including dielectric fluids for capacitors and transformers, heat transfer fluids, hydraulic fluids, lubricating and cutting oils; as additives in pesticides, paints, carbonless copy ("NCR") paper, adhesives, sealants, plastics, and reactive flame retardants; and as a fixative for microscopy. PCB mixtures are persistent organic pollutants, and have entered the environment through both use and disposal.

The skin lesions (painful bumps) occur mainly in the face, cheeks, behind the ears, armpits, groin, but in more severe cases they occur on the shoulders, chest, back, and abdomen. In advanced cases, the lesions appear also on the arms, thighs, legs, hands and feet. In some instances where the exposures are mild, chloracne may not appear until three to four weeks after toxic exposure; however, in cases of massive exposure, symptoms may appear within hours or days.

Acne Excoriee

The affected person presents with nervous, obsessive, compulsive, and habitual picking of the skin or pimple, or pulling of the hair. Up to 10% of the population is effected with some form of compulsive behavior.

What differentiates habitual picking from a true obsessive-compulsive disorder (OCD) is that OCD is done in response to a specific obsession or self-imposed rule system, i.e. "I have to wash my hands three times before taking in the laundry." Skin pickers are generally less structured. It can be ritualistic, but it is more of a mindless drive to look in the mirror for flaws, or the distracted act of pulling hangnails while doing another activity.

When this habit of picking is taken to the extreme on other parts of the body it is termed Neurotic Excoriations or "Picker's Nodules". The name explains what it is, but fails to express how painful and debilitating this disease can be. It is common for self-inflicted or self-aggravated open sores and scabs to appear all over the body. Neurotic Excoriations usually begin with a chronic fungal skin infection or Lichen Simplex Cronicus. When the scabs fail to heal in a timely manner, the patient feels an irrepressible need to pick off the scabs, feeling it is better to live with the open sores than the scabs.

Acne Due to Weather Change

Some people may notice a change in the appearance of the skin after moving to an area with a different climate. Moving from a cool to a warm climate may cause the skin to release more fluid in the form of sweat and oils in an attempt to keep the body cool. This can result in the pores of the skin becoming enlarged and shiny with the skin appearing greasy. The excess oil and sweat may clog the pores, causing blackheads and acne. Hot baths and showers cause flushing due to vasodilatation (widening of blood vessels). Individuals who prefer using warm water to open or clean pores, or to simply relax, must remember to end the process with cooler water to reverse the vasodilation.

Cold weather conditions cause vasodilatation in some people as they go from the cold outdoors into a warm indoor environment. In cold air, the heart pumps more rapidly to preserve the inner temperature and the extremities tend to cool off, however in a warm room the facial area and extremities tend to flush as the heart is still in an alert mode. Such patients are advised to wear facial masks in cold exposures, and to slowly change the temperature in their environment to help the body functions adapt to the new temperature.

Another Acne-Like Condition: Folliculitis

Folliculitis usually appears as small, white-headed pimples around one or more hair follicles, but can also appear as red bumps, or rarely as dark red scars. Superficial forms of folliculitis are most common; although they may itch, they are seldom painful, and often clear by themselves within a few days. Deep forms of folliciulis are less common; they can be more severe, may heal more slowly, and can potentially leave scars. See below for more details regarding superficial and deep forms of folliculitis.

Folliculutis has been reported to occur in persons of all races and ages. The most common causes of hair follicle damage include: friction from shaving or tight clothing, excess perspiration (which can block the follicles), inflammatory skin conditions including dermatitis and acne, skin injuries such as abrasions or surgical wounds, occlusion from plastic dressings or adhesive tape, and exposure to coal tar (common among roofers, mechanics, and oil workers). Other conditions that make patients more susceptible to folliculitis include immunosuppression, preexisting skin conditions, long-term antibiotic use, diabetes mellitus, and obesity.

Although complications of folliculitis are uncommon, they include cellulitis (swelling and tenderness caused by bacterial infection), furunculosis (recurring painful, pus-filled skin inflammation), scarring, and permanent hair loss.

Superficial Forms of Folliculitis
- **Pseudomonas folliculitis (hot tub folliculitis)**
  - o **Location.** This can occur anywhere on the body.
  - o **Appearance.** Red, round, itchy bumps, that later may develop into small pus-filled blisters (pustules), tend to form around 12-48 hours after exposure.
  - o **Cause.** The *Pseudomonas* bacteria that causes this condition thrives in a wide range of environments, including wooden hot tubs whose chlorine and pH levels are not well regulated.

- **Barber's itch**
  - o **Location.** This occurs on the beard area (face and neck) in men, and sometimes on the legs or arms in women.
  - o **Appearance.** Itchy, white, pus-filled lumps arise.
  - o **Cause.** Barber's itch appears when hair follicles that have been irritated by shaving become infected with *Staphylococcus aureus* (*Staph*) bacteria. Although *Staph* bacteria are always present on a person's skin, they generally cause problems only when they enter the body through a cut or other wound.

- **Tinea barbae**
  - o **Location.** This occurs on the beard area (face and neck) in men.

- o **Appearance.** Itchy, white bumps arise. Also, the surrounding skin also may become reddened. A more serious, inflammatory form of the infection appears as pus-filled nodules that eventually form a crust and that may occur along with swollen lymph nodes and fever.
- o **Cause.** Caused by a fungus rather than a bacterium, this type of folliculitis also develops when hair follicles become infected after being irritated by shaving.

- **Pseudofolliculitis barbae**
  - o **Location.** This occurs on the beard area (face and neck) in men.
  - o **Appearance.** Inflammation appears, and in rare cases, dark raised scars (keloid scars) develop.
  - o **Cause.** This condition develops in men with curly beards, when shaved hairs curve back into the skin.

- **Pityrosporum folliculitis**
  - o **Location.** This usually occurs on the back and chest, and sometimes on the neck, shoulders, upper arms and face.
  - o **Appearance.** Chronic, red, itchy pustules appear; this form closely resembles acne.
  - o **Cause.** Most common in young and middle-aged adults, pityrosporum folliculitis is caused by infection with a yeast-like fungus (*Malassezia furfur*), which is similar to the fungus that causes dandruff.

- **Herpetic folliculitis**
  - o **Location.** This occurs on the face area.
  - o **Appearance.** Pus-filled pimples may crust over or be surrounded by an area that is red and inflamed.

o **Cause.** This condition can develop after shaving
   through a cold sore — a small, fluid-filled blister caused
   by the herpes simplex virus — which can sometimes
   spread the herpes infection to neighboring hair follicles.

Deep Forms of Folliculitis
- **Gram-negative folliculitis**
  o **Location.** This can occur on the cheeks, chin, and
    jaw line.
  o **Appearance.** Severe acne lesions arise.
  o **Cause.** This condition sometimes develops in people
    receiving long-term antibiotic treatment for acne. Anti-
    biotics alter the normal balance of bacteria in the nose,
    leading to an overgrowth of harmful organisms (Gram-
    negative bacteria). In most people, this does not cause
    problems, and the flora in the nose returns to normal
    once antibiotics are stopped. Gram-negative bacteria
    include *Escherichia coli*, *Pseudomonas aeruginosa*,
    Serratia marcescens, and *Klebsiella* and *Proteus* spe-
    cies. In a few people, however, Gram-negative bacteria
    spread from the nose to the cheeks, chin, and jaw line,
    where they cause new and sometimes severe acne le-
    sions.

- **Boils and carbuncles**
  o **Location.** Boils typically appear on the face, neck,
    armpits, breasts, buttocks, or thighs. Carbuncles
    often occur on the back of the neck, shoulders or
    thighs, especially in older men.
  o **Appearance.** A boil usually appears suddenly as a
    painful pink or red bump about a half inch in di-
    ameter. The surrounding skin also may be red and
    swollen. Within 24 hours, the bump fills with pus. It
    grows larger and more painful for five to seven days,
    sometimes reaching golf-ball size before it develops

a yellow-white tip that finally ruptures and drains. Boils generally clear completely in about two weeks. Small boils usually heal without scarring, but a large boil may leave a scar. A carbuncle is a cluster of boils, which cause a deeper and more severe infection than a single boil. As a result, they develop and heal more slowly and are likely to leave scars.
- o **Cause.** These occur when hair follicles become deeply infected with *Staph* bacteria.

- **Eosinophilic folliculitis**
  - o **Location.** This occurs primarily on the face, and sometimes on the back or upper arms.
  - o **Appearance.** Seen primarily in HIV-infected individuals, this type of folliculitis is characterized by recurring patches of inflamed, pus-filled sores. The sores usually spread, may itch intensely, and often leave areas of hyperpigmentation (darker than normal skin) when they heal.
  - o **Cause.** The exact cause of eosinophilic folliculitis is not known, although it may involve the same yeast-like fungus responsible for pityrosporum folliculitis.

Freedom From Acne

NAET® Specialist Linda Menkhorst shared this story from her patients Lianne and Kees in the Netherlands.

We had severe food intolerance/allergy, a severe form of acne rosacea, skin problems, hay fever, bowel problems, muscle and joint problems, headache, back, and neck problems. In our deepest trouble we found during a nightly search on the internet information about NAET® with an address list of practitioners, whereby Linda Menkhorst attracted us the most.

We (my husband Kees and I) almost couldn't eat anything without allergic reactions. Only rice, courgette, carrot, broccoli, coffee, tea, water, bread, and apple jam were okay. Also medicine to treat the complaints worked the wrong way: medicines from the Western medicine, homeopathy, Chinese medicine, acupuncture, enzyme and orthomolecular therapy each gave us severe allergic reactions. We were desperate!

Linda coached us with excellence from the first phone call, and she encouraged us to treat each other at home with the result that after 16 treatments we can eat many things. A glass of milk, yogurt, normal bread instead of gluten free bread, eggs, ice cream, bakery items, tomatoes, and strawberries are just some examples of what we can eat again. Superb!

After completion of the NAET® program, not only can we eat more, but we feel ourselves much better and have much more energy, a clear skin, no hay fever, and no bowel problems, and much less headache!!!

We haven't yet treated all products we react to, but we are sure we will reach even more improvements, so after the holiday we will go on with the treatments with Linda, because she brought for us light in the deep darkness and that's what we are very grateful for!!!

Lianne and Kees

Message after awhile: *Last year this time we were deeply in trouble and didn't know what to do and if you look what we can eat now (poor weight!) and how good we feel ourselves. Really SUPERB!!! I realize myself more and more that so many "small" things are no problem anymore. We are not out of breath with hard cold wind, I have no problems with cold on my head, we have much more energy, we feel much happier and relaxed, and of course just eating deliciously and cooking with variety, even buying bread at the bakery. We have no problems when driving the car or watching TV (nausea) with moving images. We are so happy that we were treated by you with NAET®!!!*

Love, Lianne

Remarks from Linda: *There were many allergies, especially apple (which was thought to be safe), banana, nuts, zinc, heat, UV-light and of course the NAET® Basics. Stopping eating apple changed the heavily damaged skin to a perfect skin. After introducing banana the problem started again, but treatment for vitamins and fruit cleared 80% of the problem. After moving to a different area, water was again a problem. They figured out that the potassium level was different, so they treated this at home.*

(Figures 1-3 and 1-4 on the next two pages show Kees before and after NAET® treatment.)

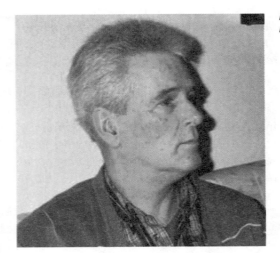

Figure 1-3. Acne rosacea before NAET®

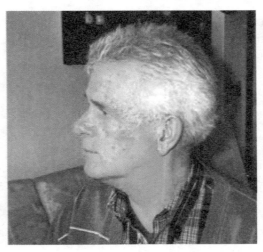

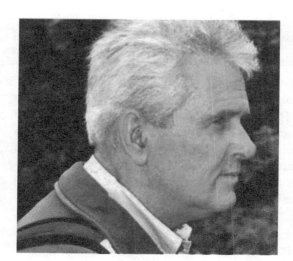

Figure 1-4. Acne rosacea after 25 NAET® treatments.

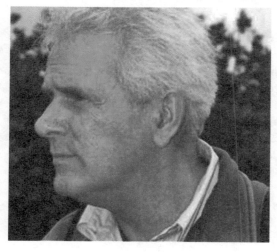

PSORIASIS

———————~~~———————

The first mention of a psoriasis-like condition was by the Greek physician Hippocrates, who lived between 460 and 377 BC. In the first century AD, a Roman author named Cornelius Celsus also wrote about psoriasis, describing it as a variation of impetigo. In the late 1700s, the English dermatologist Robert Willan recognized psoriasis as its own condition. But it was not until 1841 that the condition was given the name "psoriasis" by Viennese dermatologist Ferdinand Hebra; he was also the first to describe psoriasis as it is known today. The word was derived from the Greek word "psora" meaning "to itch".

What Are the Symptoms of Psoriasis?

Psoriasis is a chronic recurring condition that varies in severity from minor localized patches to complete body coverage. Symptoms also vary, and could include red patches, silvery white scales, small scaling spots, red pus-filled bumps, changes in fingernail or toenail appearance, and/or swollen and stiff joints. Many types of psoriasis exist, including:

Plaque Psoriasis
- **Location.** This can occur anywhere on the body, including inside the mouth, or on the genitals.
- **Appearance.** Raised areas of inflamed skin appear, covered with silvery white scaly skin that can feel itchy or sore, and can crack and bleed.

Flexural (Inverse) Psoriasis
- **Location.** This occurs in skin folds, particularly around the genitals (between the thigh and groin), the armpits, under an overweight stomach (pannus), and under the breasts.
- **Appearance.** Smooth inflamed patches of skin appear.
- **Note:** This condition is aggravated by friction and sweat, and is vulnerable to fungal infections.

Guttate Psoriasis
- **Location.** These numerous spots of psoriasis appear over large areas of the body, such as the torso, arms, legs, and scalp.
- **Appearance.** Numerous small oval (teardrop-shaped) spots appear.
- **Note.** Guttate psoriasis is associated with *Streptococcus* throat infection.

Pustular Psoriasis
- **Location.** This can be localized, commonly to the hands and feet (palmoplantar pustulosis), or generalized with widespread patches occurring randomly anywhere on the body.
- **Appearance.** Raised bumps appear, and are filled with noninfectious pus (pustules). The skin under and surrounding pustules is red and tender.

Nail Psoriasis
- **Location.** This occurs on fingernails and toenails.
- **Appearance.** Nail psoriasis produces a variety of changes in the appearance, including discoloration under the nail plate, pitting of the nails, lines going across the nails, thickening of the skin under the nails, and the loosening (onycholysis) and crumbling of the nails.

Erythrodermic Psoriasis
- **Location.** This occurs on most of the body surface.
- **Appearance.** Widespread inflammation and exfoliation of the skin occurs, and may be accompanied by severe itching, swelling, and pain.
- **Note.** It often results from an exacerbation of unstable plaque psoriasis, particularly following the abrupt withdrawal of systemic treatment. This form of psoriasis can be fatal, as the extreme inflammation and exfoliation disrupt the body's ability to regulate temperature and the skin's ability to perform barrier functions.

Psoriatic Arthritis
- **Location.** This is most common in the joints of the fingers and toes, but can affect any joint including the hips, knees, and spine (spondylitis).
- **Appearance.** Joint and connective tissue inflammation causes pain in the affected areas. In the fingers or toes, this can result in a sausage-shaped swelling.
- **Note.** Approximately 10-15% of people who have psoriasis also have psoriatic arthritis.

What Causes Psoriasis?

The cause of psoriasis is not known. Genetic predisposition may be a factor: about one third of people with this condition report a family history of psoriasis; and, studies reported in the July 2005 issue of the *Journal of the American Academy of Dermatology* suggest that in twins, there is a 67% chance of developing psoriasis if an identical twin has psoriasis, but only a 18% chance of developing psoriasis if a nonidentical (fraternal) twin has psoriasis. Several other factors are thought to aggravate psoriasis, including stress, excessive alcohol consumption, and smoking. Individuals with psoriasis may suffer from depression and loss of self-esteem. As such, quality of life is an important factor in evaluating the severity of the disease.

How Common Is Psoriasis?

Psoriasis affects both sexes equally and can occur at any age, although it most commonly appears for the first time between the ages of 15 and 25 years.

Statistics show that approximately 2-3% (7 million people) in the United States have symptoms of psoriasis. A survey conducted by the National Psoriasis Foundation found that 2.1% of adult Americans have symptoms of psoriasis, among whom 35% have moderate to severe psoriasis.

Onset before age 40 usually indicates a greater genetic susceptibility and a more severe or recurrent course of psoriasis.

What Are the Complications of Psoriasis?

Depending on the severity of the condition, individuals may experience significant physical discomfort and some disability. Itching and pain can interfere with basic functions, such as self-care, walking, and sleep. Plaques on hands and feet can prevent individuals from working in certain occupations, playing sports, caring for family members, or taking care of a home. The frequency of medical care is costly and can interfere with an employment or school schedule. Individuals with psoriasis may also feel self-conscious about their appearance and have a poor self-image. Psychological distress can lead to significant depression and social isolation. Quality of life can be impaired due to these reasons.

Freedom From Psoriasis

Maxine Poe shared this story about how she finally became free from psoriasis.

I have suffered from psoriasis for the past 43 years. It started when I was 29 years old, soon after I began working as an office secretary with an aircraft company in Orange County, California. I also suffered from frequent muscle spasms, backaches, and headaches. I tried various therapies and medications. I tried acupuncture and a variety of homeopathic remedies too. Nothing gave me significant relief. Finally I was referred to a chiropractor. Regular chiropractic treatments three times weekly gave me great relief from my headaches and backaches for a few hours after each adjustment.

My psoriasis, dry skin, and white scaly skin continued until I was 72 years old. Then I met Dr. Devi at my chiropractor's office. In fact he introduced her to me, and suggested that I try her new treatment for my dry skin. I thought, "What's there to lose?" So I decided to take her special acupuncture/acupressure treatments.

With her kinesiological testing she determined that my skin problem was coming from ingesting milk products. She told me to avoid milk and milk products until she cleared the allergic reaction to them. I told her that I haven't used milk in forty years ever since my chiropractor advised me to stay away from milk to improve my dry skin. I drank black coffee ever since. She tested again and said that I was using milk products five days a week, probably as cottage cheese. As she mentioned cottage cheese, I let out a cry. How dumb I was! Of course, I was taking a banana and cottage cheese for lunch every day to work, and ate it regularly. Even after retirement I continued with my custom of eating a healthy lunch – cottage cheese and banana. Somehow my brain didn't associate cottage cheese with milk product.

Dr. Devi advised me to stay away from all types of cheeses, butter, yogurt, cookies, and cakes, until I was treated for milk products. Just by avoiding the cottage cheese I noticed a great difference. My frequent migraines were reduced, my skin became less dry, and my psoriasis began disappearing. Then I was treated with NAET® for calcium mix, milk mix, and cheese mix. When I completed the treatments for milk products, my skin became normal.

After 43 years of constant struggle with my health, finally I am blessed to enjoy a few years without headaches and psoriasis. I am 76 years old now. For the past four years I have been free of my psoriasis and headaches. Thank you Dr. Devi for developing this unique treatment.

CANDIDIASIS

Candidiasis is an infection caused by a microscopic fungi or yeast in the *Candida* family. There are more than 20 species of *Candida*, the most common being *Candida albicans* (which causes oral "thrush" and vaginal yeast infections).

What Are the Symptoms of Candidiasis?

- **Location.** *Candida* infections can affect the skin, mouth, esophagus (swallowing tube), and genitals. Skin infections commonly occur in warm moist body areas, such as armpits. Usually the skin effectively blocks yeast, but any breakdown or cuts in the skin may allow this organism to penetrate. Skin areas typically affected in babies include the mouth and diaper areas. In adults, oral yeast infections become more common with increased age. Adults can also have yeast infections around dentures, under the breast and lower abdomen, fingernails or toenails, beneath other skin folds, and in genital areas. Most of these *Candida* infections are superficial and clear up easily with treatment. Rarely, the yeast infection may spread throughout the body. In systemic *Candida* disease, up to 75% of people may die. Even common mouth and vaginal yeast infections can cause critical illness and can be more resistant to normal treatment. Yeast infections that return may be a sign of more serious diseases such as diabetes, leukemia, or HIV/AIDS.
- **Appearance.** Symptoms of candidiasis depend on the part of the body affected. The most common symptoms are as follows:
  - o **Cutaneous candidiasis.** Candidiasis can appear like many of the other skin conditions described above,

such as rash, acne, athlete's foot, chronic toenail and fingernail fungus, ridging or discoloration, dandruff, eczema (dermatitis, skin rashes), hair loss, hives, jock itch, rectal itching, dry skin, flaking skin, and skin discoloration. The skin could also feel like ants crawling on it ("crawling skin").

o **Oral candidiasis.** Some of the general symptoms of oral "thrush" include burning pain in the mouth or throat, altered taste (especially when eating spicy or sweet foods), and difficulty swallowing. Oral candidiasis appears as white or pinkish-red blotches on the tongue, gums, the sides or roof of the mouth, and the back of the throat. Sometimes, oral candidiasis can cause the corners of the mouth to become chapped, cracked, and sore (angular cheilitis). Dryness of the mouth and chronic dental problems are also seen in people with oral candidiasis.

o **Esophageal candidiasis.** This type of candidiasis occurs deep down in the throat and cannot always be seen by looking into the mouth. Symptoms include sore throat with pain and difficulty upon swallowing, or brown colored mucus in the back of the throat. It can also cause chest pain. Esophageal candidiasis is much more common in HIV-infected individuals due to their suppressed immune systems.

o **Vaginal candidiasis.** The most obvious symptom of vaginal yeast infections is a thick white discharge that resembles cottage cheese. It can also cause itching and burning in or around the vagina, as well as tenderness and rash on the labia (outer lips of the vagina). Women with HIV infection are more likely to experience recurrent vaginal yeast infections than women who are not infected with HIV. Symptoms include severe itching, burning, and soreness, irritation of the vagina and/or vulva, and a whitish or whitish-gray discharge, often with a curd-like appearance. Many women mistake the symptoms of the more common bacterial vaginosis for a yeast infection. In a 2002 study published in the journal *Obstetrics and Gynecology*, only 33% of women who were self treating for a yeast infection actually had a yeast infection; instead they had either bacterial vaginosis or a mixed-type infection.

o   **Male genital symptoms.** In men, symptoms of candidiasis include red patchy sores near the head of the penis or on the foreskin. The sores may feel irritated and itchy, and sometimes they will burn as well.

What Causes Candidiasis?

Candida species are a part of normal flora, so the yeast organisms are always present in all people, but are usually prevented from "overgrowth" by other naturally occurring microorganisms ("native bacteria"). If native bacteria are decreased, *Candida* can multiply and cause symptoms. There are over 20 species of *Candida*; the most common is *Candida albicans*.

Factors that can decrease native bacteria can include:

•   **Antibiotics.** The most common factor contributing to candidiasis is the use of broad-spectrum antibiotics, which decrease the number of normal flora and permit the overgrowth of *Candida* in the body.

•   **Hormonal changes.** Increased estrogen levels (associated with estrogen-containing birth control pills, pregnancy, Hormone Replacement Therapy, or infertility treatments) cause changes in the vaginal environment that make it perfect for fungal growth and nourishment.

•   **Weakened immune system.** Infections of any kind are more common when the immune system is weakened, such as in HIV infection or diabetes, or with certain medications such as steroids or anticancer drugs. A baby's young immune system is vulnerable to infection; a baby can contract candidiasis from an infected mother, either while passing through the birth canal, or through breast-feeding.

- **Poor diet.** Some people develop candidiasis due to their poor diet. *Candida* overgrowth occurs in the body when food is not properly digested, resulting in poor absorption and assimilation of nutrients. Poor assimilation of nutrients leads to a weak immune system and poor circulation of energy, building up the waste products in the body, mainly in the gut. This disturbs the intestinal flora. Yeast and *Candida* multiply by the millions to ferment the waste buildup in the gut, and then to travel to other parts of the body.

- **Poor energy circulation.** This is caused by several factors, including an allergy to food products, leading to blockages in the energy meridians; diseases (diabetes, chronic infections, leukemia, cancer); lack of production of essential gastric juices and digestive enzymes; use of antibiotics or birth control pills; treatment with radiation or chemotherapy; hormone imbalance; exposure to toxic chemicals; nutritional deficiencies, such as a high carbohydrate diet, poor eating habits, foods that irritate the mucous membrane of the small intestine (carbonated drinks), not drinking enough water to flush out the system, and poor personal hygiene.

- According to NAET® theory, allergies are the cause of most yeast and *Candida* infections. Individuals may be allergic to various substances: food, drinks, rice, wheat, corn, grains, sugar and sugar products, refined starches, coffee, chocolate, spices, deep fried foods, acidic foods, fruits, moldy food, wool, cotton, silk, polyester, acrylic, acetate, or other fabrics, silica, salt, ocean water, rainwater, heat, humidity, vegetables, nuts, processed foods, food colorings, food additives, food preservatives, vitamins, herbal supplements, hormone supplements, other drugs, sanitary napkins, tampons, cotton crotches of underwear, pantyhose, toilet paper, body soap, detergent, skin creams, spouses, partners, saliva, semen, vaginal mucus, other body secretions, bed linen, plastic bath toys and accessories, and pets. (See Chapter 2 for more information on allergies.)

How Common Is Candidiasis?

In the United States, statistics indicate that over 50% of healthy individuals develop symptoms of candidiasis; in most cases, symptoms are superficial and resolve completely. Nearly 15% of patients with immunocompromising disease develop systemic candidiasis.

Males and females are affected equally by most forms of *Candida* species. *Candida albicans* is the most common cause of oral thrush and esophagitis.

All ages are affected by candidiasis. Newborn babies commonly have perianal infection (diaper rash) and oral thrush. In adults, oral and gastrointestinal candidiasis occur more often with increased age; the elderly are most often affected.

Freedom From Candidiasis

Janet Johnson from Riverside, California, shared her story about how she finally became free from her candidiasis.

I have been a patient of Dr. Devi for three years. When I first started the allergy treatments, I was in pretty bad condition. My health deteriorated 12 years ago when I came down with chronic fatigue. I had constant sinus infections for years, and the antibiotics I took gave me Candida *infection. I suffered from severe systemic candidiasis for years. I had frequent headaches, body pain, bladder infections, and a fever for over a year and a half. My uterus was detaching and I had large cysts on my ovaries. I was exhausted all the time. I saw many doctors during the past 12 years and everyone of them diagnosed my condition as simply an overgrowth of Candida and yeast. I went through various detox programs and took the mercury out of my teeth, tried to eat healthy at home, spent thousands of dollars and suffered the pain and agony every day, in spite of everything I was doing to feel better. I suffered from severe insomnia, too. Doctors could offer only drugs, surgery, and exercise recommendations. But when you have to rest just to get energy to go upstairs in your house, it is pretty hard to find the energy to exercise. I tried everything that I knew to get well, including a healthy diet, rest, and acupuncture with Chinese herbal teas, at great expense. This helped some, but not permanently. Little did I know I was allergic to everything I was eating and drinking, along with the environmental pollutions. Previous allergy testing using conventional methods only showed environmental allergies. I was 38 years old and I thought my life was over.*

After I started treatment with Dr. Devi my health has steadily improved. It took about three months of Basic treatments for the chronic fatigue and Candida, after which I noticed a change. When I was treated for minerals, the cysts on my ovaries disappeared and my uterus reattached. A sonogram and examination confirmed and showed everything was as normal once again.

I still receive treatments once in awhile. But I have a life again. After 15 years of gap, I started working on a regular job. All my infections are long gone and headaches are rare. I exercise and I know I will live a long life in health and with energy.

I learned to test everything before I buy. At first I thought that testing everything as Dr. Devi had suggested was a hassle. I soon realized that is was the only way to stay healthy without al-

lergic reactions. We cannot buy the same product everyday. The cultivation of the products, the fertilizers, the pesticide contents, the preparation, the packaging, the additives, etc. change in the products even if we buy the same name-brands. Our bodies can perceive the change as an allergen and react to the item causing new reactions or bringing back the previous reactions. Testing before buying or consuming gives us the ability to screen the reactions before they control us.

Thank God for Dr. Devi and NAET® treatment. This is a real and permanent solution for any health problem.

ATHLETE'S FOOT

Athlete's foot (tinea pedis) is a common persistent infection of the foot caused by a microscopic fungus that lives on dead tissue of the hair, toenails, and outer skin layers. The infection is transmitted from person to person from anywhere there is high potential for contact with the fungus; the infection enters the body through a cut or abrasion on the bottom (plantar surface) of the foot. These fungi thrive in warm, moist environments such as shoes, stockings, and the floors of public showers, locker rooms, swimming pools, gymnasiums, and other areas where people share facilities or walk barefoot. These parasitic fungi grow anywhere in the body that is fairly moist and unexposed to sunlight or air.

Skin infections cause raised, circular pimples or blisters that resemble the lesions caused by ringworm. The infections are named for the part of the body they infect; therefore, tinea pedis refers to an infection of the feet.

What Are the Symptoms of Athlete's Foot?

Common symptoms include persistent itching of the skin on the sole of the foot or between the toes (often the fourth and fifth toes). As the infection progresses, the skin grows soft and the center of the infection becomes inflamed and sensitive to the touch. Gradually, the edges of the infected area become milky white and the skin begins to peel. A slight watery discharge also may be present.

Tinea pedis is inflammatory or vesicular, in which a series of raised bumps or ridges develops under the skin on the bottom of the foot, typically in the region of the ends of the long bones in the foot. Itching can be intense. People with acute tinea infections can develop similar symptoms on their hands, typically on the palms. This reaction, also known as tineas manuum, is an immune system response to the antibodies that fight the fungal infection.

Tinea infections may disappear spontaneously, or can persist for years.

What Causes Athlete's Foot?

This condition is caused by dermatophytes, a group of parasitic fungi that infects the skin. Dermatophytes cause infections of the skin, hair, and nails, because they feed on the keratin found in these parts of the body.

Some of these infections are also known as ringworm or tinea. Toenail and fingernail infections are referred to as onychomycosis. Dermatophytes usually do not invade living tissues, but colonize the outer layer of the skin.

How Common Is Athlete's Foot?

Athlete's foot is a very common type of fungal infection. Statistics indicate that about 10% of the population will have this condition at any given time. Athlete's foot is most common in teenage to middle-age men, and in people with compromised immune systems.

Freedom From Athlete's Foot

Mike Salzman from Los Angeles, Califorinia, shared this story.

I suffered from athlete's foot for many years. I had to visit my podiatrist once a week. I also took extra care of my foot on my own. I spent hours soaking my feet in the saline water, drying them, applying castor oil packs, egg white poultice, etc. to get relief of the pain caused from athlete's foot. (Athlete's foot can be very painful sometimes.) Then I came to Dr. Devi for my headaches. She treated me for all the Basic allergens. I had five NAET® treatments on five different days for grain mix. When I passed the treatment for grain mix, I noticed my feet were cleared of the athlete's foot problem. I don't spend much time on my foot care anymore. NAET® is amazing! Thank you Dr. Devi.

BALDNESS AND HAIR LOSS

What Are the Symptoms?

Hair loss (also called alopecia) involves the state of lacking hair where it often grows. The severity and nature of hair loss can vary greatly:

- **Alopecia areata.** This involves the loss of hair from one area, usually a spot on the head; this includes:
  o **Alopecia androgenetica**, also known as male and female pattern baldness, which involves receding hairline and/or bald patch on the top of the head;
  o **Alopecia cicatricial**, which involves localized or diffuse hair loss on the head, and can be associated with severe itching, burning, and pain, redness, scaling, changes in pigmentation, or pustules.
- **Alopecia totalis.** This involves the loss of all hair on the head.
- **Alopecia universalis.** This involves the loss of all hair on the head and the body.

Temporary loss of hair can occur in areas where sebaceous cysts are present for one to several weeks. Permanent hair loss can occur when the hair follicles are destroyed. Onset of hair loss can begin as early as the end of puberty (mostly due to genetic factors).

What Causes Hair Loss?

Hair loss can be caused by one or more factors, including:

- Genetics (family history)
- Autoimmune disorders (e.g., with alopecia cicatricial, which may occur with lupus erythematosus, lichen plano pilaris, folliculitis decalvans)
- Hormonal deficiencies or imbalances
- Hypothyroidism (especially thinning of the outer third of the eyebrows)
- Nutritional deficiencies, such as Vitamin A or D
- Fungal infection
- Traumas such as chemotherapy, childbirth, major surgery, poisoning, and severe stress (e.g., with Telogen effluvium alopecia)
- Pulling on hair with excessive force, such as with cornrows or ponytails (e.g., Traction alopecia)
- Skin tumors (skin outgrowths or cancers)
- Allergy to the patient's own hormones (e.g., thyroid or adrenal hormones), or to other substances (e.g., hat, water, shampoo, hair creams, conditioner, hair dye, cotton towels)

How Common Is Hair Loss?

The most common form of hair loss is male pattern baldness. Statistics show that this is responsible for 95% of hair loss in men; by age 35, 66% of men have some hair loss, and by age 50 about 85% of men have significant hair loss.

What Are the Complications of Hair Loss?

Psychological effects vary widely in people who experience hair loss. Some people adapt to the change comfortably, while others have severe problems relating to anxiety, depression, social phobia, body image, and in some cases, identity change.

Counselling and family therapy can help families to cope with these psychological problems if they arise.

Freedom From Hair Loss

Effrain Habib from Los Angeles, California, shared this story.

I suffered from severe hair loss for the past three years. I almost became bald. My father and uncles became bald by the time they reached 50. I was only 27 years old then. I was very worried. I even thought of going for hair transplantation. Then I read in the Orange County newspaper about this new revolutionary treatment called NAET®. I immediately called for an appointment and began treatments. I was treated five times a week by Dr. Devi for all Basic allergens. Then I was treated for other allergens from my surroundings, like tap water, cotton towel, shampoo, hair conditioner, soap, plastics, a hair brush, and some of them in combinations with hormones. She also put me on Chinese herbs. In about six months time my hair stopped falling. After completing NAET® I waited patiently for about nine months, checking daily for any sign of hair growth. Dr. Devi had warned me that it might take over a year to see any new growth. It took only about nine months before I saw the sign of new hair growth. Now I have normal hair growth. In the meantime I practiced my muscle testing skills to check for allergies. Now I check every product I buy for my hair before using it. I am very happy to report that I continue to enjoy my normal hair without having to worry about the hair loss.

CHAPTER 2

WHAT TYPES OF ALLERGIES TRIGGER SKIN DISORDERS?

Taking a Closer Look: Categories of Allergens

OVERVIEW

*P*eople have been suffering from various skin disorders for a long time, probably since the beginning of human existence. However, no one knows the actual cause of many skin disorders. Most health care practitioners identify skin disorders according to the patient's symptoms. Symptom-oriented treatments help keep patients calm, and work very well most of the time. When symptoms are gone, the doctor and patient are happy. However, no one looks for the original trigger that started the symptoms. So, at times when symptomatic treatments do not work, the doctor is puzzled, and the patient is confused and disappointed. In today's world this is a frequent scenario.

Using NAET® theory and after seeing hundreds of people with various illnesses and skin problems, this author can confidently and boldly state that allergies are the cause of most patients' skin problems. Over the past 25 years, this author has proven the NAET® theory that there is always an allergic factor behind each and every illness. When an allergen is removed or eliminated through NAET® desensitization methods (discussed in Chapter 4), the original health problems (eczema or other skin disorders) are reduced or completely eliminated. Individuals who suffer from eczema and other skin disorders are sensitive to foods, environmental substances, and chemical substances from their surroundings. They also have very fragile emotions. When they live with all of these allergies, an energy disturbances in lung, large intestine, heart, small intestine, spleen, stomach, liver and/or gallbladder meridians (see Chapter 3) results in continued suffer-ring from eczema, acne, or other skin problems, in spite of vari-ous treatments including prescription and nonprescription medi-cations.

A person can be allergic to anything, including: foods, drinks, prescription drugs, over-the-counter drugs, illicit drugs, herbs, vitamins, tap water, purified water, rain water, clothing, jewelry, precious stones, heavy metals, ice, cold, heat, wind, work materi-als, his/her own body secretions, body organs, chemicals, form-aldehyde, office and building materials, paints, toxins from the environment, toxins produced internally due to faulty digestion, pressed wood, plant enzymes, terpenes, phenolics, aldehydes, acetaldehydes, synthetically made additives, silica, silicone, la-tex, plastics, synthetic fibers and products, pollens, grasses, trees, wood, house plants, imitation plants, sand, rock, and ocean wa-ter. Undiagnosed allergies can produce symptoms, illnesses, and even chronic diseases, including chronic eczema, acne, candidiasi (yeast infection), or other skin ailments.

By learning the simple NAET® testing procedures (see Chap-ter 3), anyone, professional or public, can learn to recognize vari-ous allergens and their associated ill-health conditions. This will help the person suffering from chronic symptoms to begin seek-ing the appropriate diagnostic studies, and to pursue proper health care as needed. When the diagnosis is correct, problems become less frightening than an uncertain explanation. Determining the right *trigger* for the skin disorder is the first step in diagnosing the condition accurately.

Common allergens are generally classified into nine general categories, based primarily on the method in which they are contacted, rather than the symptoms they produce. These categories of allergens are:

1. Inhalants
2. Ingestants
3. Contactants
4. Injectants
5. Infectants
6. Physical agents
7. Genetic factors
8. Molds and fungi
9. Psychogenic causes

INHALANTS

Inhalants are those allergens that are contacted through the nose, throat, and bronchial tubes. Examples of inhalants include: microscopic spores of certain grasses, flowers, pollens, powders, smoke, cosmetics, dust, dust mites, flour from grains, perfumes, smoke from a fireplace, burning wood, pollution in the air, flower fragrance, cooking fragrance, fermented foods, body odor, body secretions of self or others, smell of decayed substance, smell of stale food, smell from animal droppings when visiting an animal farm, or even the smell of carpets, bed, bed linen, pillows, fabric covered sofas and other furniture, draperies, or car seats.

Sometimes, these smells can produce watery eyes, runny nose, coughing, bronchial spasms, asthma, fainting episodes, or even hives and eczema. The smell receptors and spleen meridian (see Chapter 3 for more information on meridians) have become the weakest tissue in this group and they have become supersensitive to natural smells from the environment.

In the case of dust mites, which accumulate in carpets, pillows, and beds, it is easy to frequently wash pillows and bed linens to kill the dust mites and their eggs. However, beds are not easy to wash frequently. Beds can be completely covered with thick plastics. Then the beds should be protected with mattress covers and bed sheets, which can be washed regularly. Air purifiers and room purifiers or humidifiers can help clean the bedrooms. Whenever possible, curtains and windows should be opened for fresh air circulation. Sunlight can also help kill dust mites.

One of my seven-year-old female patients complained of severe itching, hives, eventually whole body rashes as soon as she was put to bed at night. She woke up with severe itching and often with asthma around 3:00 a.m. every morning for the last four years. For the first two years she suffered the itching. Then her parents took her to the doctor. After trying different treatments for itching and rashes without getting any results for the next two more years, she was referred to us by one of her friends. Her history pointed towards something in the bed causing the problem. She was treated with NAET® for the bed linens, pillow cases, etc., but she continued to have itching. Her mother said she slept with a teddy bear bed pillow every night, so she was asked to bring her pillow. She was allergic to the pillow. After the treatment with NAET® for her teddy bear, her asthma and itching reduced. Her teddy bear was also sent for cleaning. When it returned after cleaning, she stopped having any more itching in the bed.

Another patient suffered from chronic cough, fatigue, insomnia, and whole body itching for over four years. She was allergic to her carpet. She said the carpet was about 10 years old. She did not have the cough for six years. She could not understand why her cough and itching started only after six years. She was not convinced that carpet could be the cause for her cough. So, we did not treat her for the carpet. Instead, she was advised to replace the old carpet. We wanted to show her how much she was affected by the carpet and just by avoiding the suspected allergen how much improvement she could receive. She decided to do that before receiving any treatment with NAET® for the carpet. When the carpet people came in and removed the carpet she said there were millions of black eggs and tiny worms crawling under the carpet. She decided to put ceramic tiles in the bedroom instead of the carpet. A week after replacing the carpet she returned to my office. She was completely free from her cough for the whole week. But when she returned to work, her cough returned. She had carpets in her office. Since the allergies to carpet and carpet mites were left untreated, even though she was not coughing in her house, she was bothered by other places with carpets. She could not ask everyone to replace their carpets with tiles. So this time she was desperate and wanted to be treated for the carpet allergy. Of course, she had to be treated for the NAET® Basic allergies first before she was treated for the carpet, mites, dust, and dust mites. After successful completion of these treatments she said none of them, including new or old carpets, dust or dust mites, or dusty areas, make her itch or cough anymore. But she said that she makes sure she wears slippers while walking on carpets just in case some of the worms from beneath the carpets decide to crawl into her clothes without her knowledge. She did not want to take any more chances.

Another young patient broke out in rashes and hives every morning upon awakening. She was allergic to the smell of the coffee brewing in the house.

Another young lady began itching and scratching every time she visited a movie house. She was allergic to the smell of the popcorn that was so unavoidable in the movie house. Finally she stopped going for movies until after she was treated with NAET® for the smell of popcorn.

INGESTANTS

Ingestants are allergens that enter the body through the mouth and find their way into the gastrointestinal tract.

Allergy to Foods, Drinks, and Nutrients

Various foods and drinks, food additives, coloring, condiments, drugs, chewing gums, vitamin supplements, etc. can trigger eczema in sensitive people. Deficiency of filaggrin, a specific protein for skin health, also causes skin problems. Duhring's Disease, which causes intense itching and typically symmetrical rash on arms, thighs, knees, and back, is directly related to celiac disease, and can often be put into remission with appropriate diet. Lack of essential vitamins, minerals, proteins, fatty acids, or other nutrients can cause itching and symmetrical rash on arms, thighs, knees, and back due to nutritional deficiencies. Nutritional deficiencies can result from poor food intake or poor food absorption and assimilation, due to allergies to those nutritional elements.

Ingestant allergies are difficult to diagnose, because the allergic responses are often delayed (from several minutes to several days), making the direct association between cause and effect unclear. This is not to say that an immediate response is not possible. Some people can react violently in seconds after they consume an allergen. In extreme cases, one has to only touch or come near the allergen to signal the central nervous system that it is about to be poisoned, resulting in symptoms that are peculiar to that particular patient. Usually, more violent reactions are observed with ingested allergens than with other types of allergens. Processed or unprocessed tree nuts, eggs, milk, fish, herbs, herbal teas, spices, and other ingestants can cause immediate or delayed reactions, giving rise to various health problems.

One NAET® Specialist, Marilyn Chernoff, N.D., Ph.D., M.Ed., from New Mexico, U.S.A., shared this story with photos (Figures 2-1 and 2-2) from her patient, Sasha, whose allergy to salt caused hand eczema. *Thank you so much, for clearing my very bad hurting knuckles. I am 10 years old and this treatment was hard because I could only eat fruits, vegetables, and chicken. I mean I couldn't eat any of the Christmas party snacks and I wasn't happy. I was on the salt treatment. My friends and teachers were worried about my hands because they were bloody and cracky. After the treatment I was glad I didn't eat the brownies or cupcakes, or drink the root beer, because my hands didn't hurt at all. I remembered that I could only drink distilled water and could only touch distilled water. I brought my own water to school. Right after the 25 hours of the treatment, my knuckles didn't hurt anymore. Everyone noticed how much better they looked after one day. Now it's three days after the treatment, and my brother and I think it's amazing. Thank you very much, Dr. Chernoff. NAET® is neat.*

Another NAET® Specialist, Yumie Saito, R.N., D.C. from Tokyo, Japan, shared this story of her three-and-a-half-year-old patient with atopic dermatitis. *In my office, I have seen a few patients with atopic dermatitis, however, most of them were already treated by corticosteroids before they came to me. Usually the patients went to dermatologists first and they were medicated with cortisone, etc. to reduce or control the inflammation. But if their dermatitis was caused from allergies, there was a good chance that the patients were allergic to the medication that they took to reduce the condition. Such allergic patients often got severe dermatitis probably due to their allergies to the drug, cortisone. (Such cases are often very difficult to treat successfully.) I am going to present a case of atopic dermatitis here. This patient was not seen by any dermatologist nor treated by cortisone or any other drugs. Therefore I can report this case purely from an NAET® point of view.*

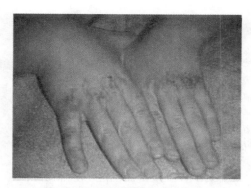

Figure 2-1. Hand eczema before NAET® treatment.

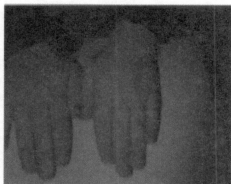

Figure 2-2. Hand eczema after NAET® treatment.

History: At the age of one month, this patient did not open his eyes due to lots of mucus in the eyes. At the age of two months he began developing eczema, and soon his entire body was covered with eczema. (See Figure 2-3.) His mother did not take him to a dermatologist for this condition; instead she brought him to me.

Treatment: On March 19, 2005, this three-and-a-half-month old baby was brought to my office by his mother, who was also my patient. This young boy presented with atopic dermatitis. His whole body, including head, face, neck, hand, back, leg and feet were covered with eczema. According to his mother, the skin eruptions gradually started to appear at the age of two months. His mother reported that he was very irritable and crying from itching and scratching his body most of the time. During the three-month check-up at the well-baby clinic, the pediatrician noticed the eczema. He found it difficult to locate a clear site to administer the vaccination because the whole body was covered with eczema.

I immediately started NAET® treatments on the child, beginning with brain-body balance formula (BBF) on the first visit, followed by treatment for breast milk three times on the following visits. When he finally passed treatment for the breast milk, I tested him by question-response technique (QRT) to find the most beneficial treatment of that day in order to give him some relief from his discomfort. QRT revealed allergy to grain mix, wheat mix, and soybean mix, and I continued to treat him accordingly.

Gradually his symptoms began to diminish. The oozing of pus stopped and scabs began forming. During his four-month well-baby check-up, his pediatrician highly recommended that he be treated with corticosteroids, however, the child's mother decided to continue the NAET® treatments in my office instead. She kept his hands in mittens all the time in order to prevent him from scratching himself and causing any bleeding.

The next treatment priority was to treat soy sauce twice, miso (fermented soybean) three times, yeast mix five times, egg mix twice, and mold mix three times. By the first week of June, 2005, upon completing the above treatments, the child stopped itching completely. His skin began to appear somewhat normal. During that time he was taken to the pediatrician for his DPT immunization. The mother was very happy to note that the pediatrician could not find much skin abnormality on the child that he had noticed on his previous visit. This time he had no problem to locate an appropriate site for inoculation.

In August 2005, he was bitten by mosquitoes at various sites on his body and the sites became red and swollen. I treated him

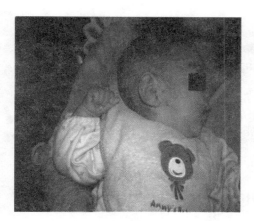

Figure 2-3. Three-and-a-half-month-old infant with atopic dermatitis, before NAET® treatment.

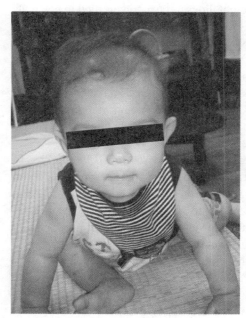

Figure 2-4. Three-and-a-half-month-old infant with atopic dermatitis, after NAET® treatment.

In September, I started to treat rice with various combinations such as stomach, skin, base, leukotriene, IgE, and emotions for preparing him for weaning from breast milk.

Result: At this time his skin disorder is totally gone. By the end of September 2005, he received a total of 51 NAET® treatments and ever since he has remained without skin problems (see Figure 2-4).

Allergy to Drugs

In 1996, one hundred eight thousand Americans died in hospitals from adverse reactions to FDA-approved drugs properly administered by licensed medical professionals, as reported by the *Journal of the American Medical Association*. In the same year, 2.2 million Americans had adverse reactions to FDA-approved drugs. This report also indicated that adverse drug reactions affect a far greater number of hospital patients than was previously thought and may rank as high as the fourth leading cause of death in the United States.

Individuals who are allergic to foods can also be allergic to drugs. Without realizing the status of their allergy, drugs are taken by the allergic patients causing hives, urticaria, itching, eczema, edema, anaphylaxis, and/or death. If the individuals are not allergic to the drugs they ingest or inject, they will not produce any adverse symptoms. Drug reaction usually causes hives, itching and eczema in sensitive individuals.

Toxic Overload in the Body

Overeating, constipation, improper elimination can cause food stasis in the body and overload of toxic food in the colon can trigger eczema.

CONTACTANTS

Contactants produce their effect by direct contact with the skin. Contact dermatitis is allergic in origin; there are two types: allergic contact dermatitis resulting from a delayed reaction to some allergen, and irritant contact dermatitis resulting from direct reaction to a chemical or solvent. Some substances act both as allergen and irritant. Other substances cause a problem when they combine with another agent.

Contactants that commonly cause reactions include the well-known poison oak, poison ivy, and poison sumac, as well as cats, dogs, rabbits, wood furniture, wood cabinets, ornamental iron works, iron skillets, utensils, trees, grasses, weeds, pollens, flowers, early morning dew, natural fabrics (such as cotton, silk, and wool), jute, feathers, herbs, various types of plant oils, petroleum jelly, lanolin hand creams, ceramics, dirt, insects, animal dander, epithelials (skin cells), animal droppings, human hair, rocks, stones, precious stones (such as diamonds, emeralds, and crystals), spring water, drinking water, silica, silicone, glass, sand on the beach, ocean water, ocean air, crude oil, and products made from crude oil.

Allergic reactions to contactants can be different in each person, and may include: eczema, acne, dry skin, itching, boils, ulcers, skin cancer, skin rashes, sneezing attacks, swelling of the body. Patients with contactant allergies also often suffer from depression, panic attacks, nervousness, queasy stomach, unexplained fear, feelings of insecurity, helplessness, diarrhea, abdominal cramps, internal tremors, insomnia, fibromyalgia, general fatigue, poor appetite, and weight loss.

Allergens and Irritants

Allergic Contact Dermatitis

This condition can occur by direct contact with the allergen. For example, housewife's eczema or allergic eczema can develop from contact with fabrics, cosmetics, dishwashing soap, dish scrubber, housecleaning chemicals, gloves, etc. Allergic contact dermatitis develops when the body's immune system reacts against a substance that is in contact with the skin. The allergic reaction often develops over a period of time through repeated contact with the substance (delayed reaction). For example, an allergic reaction may occur to nickel, which is often found in earrings, belt buckles, and buttons. Reactions can also occur after contact with other substances such as perfumes and rubber. To prevent repeated reactions, it is best for to prevent contact with anything that is known to cause a rash in that person. Contact dermatitis is curable if the offending item is detected, avoided, and (preferably) treated with NAET® desensitization.

The following story from the author's private practice demonstrates how contact dermatitis even from an unknown contactant can be helped with NAET® desensitization treatments. *A 28-year-old housewife came to see me for her hand eczema. She had her hands inside cotton gloves. She wore cotton gloves whenever she left her house. She was embarrassed to show her hands to anyone. According to this patient, she had suffered from severe hand eczema for the past four years. She had tried to avoid all chemicals in the house. She had help with housecleaning, so she did not have to do any work with her hands. She took off the gloves so that I could examine her hands, revealing that she had weeping eczema on both palms and some dry eczema on the back of both hands. She also had a couple of deep fissures inside the palm. Upon NAET® testing, peanuts were found to be the causative agent for her hand eczema. To my puzzlement, she said that she never ate peanuts, and she had not touched peanuts for years. In fact, she hated all nuts, especially peanuts, since she was a child. Her husband never liked peanuts either. So they never brought peanuts or any other nuts in the house at all.*

If done correctly, people cannot fool NAET®. NAET® theory believes that the brain never lies. My further NAET® testing revealed that she had been touching the peanut or peanut product early in the morning, three or four times weekly, for the last four years. She was not eating it herself. When I told her my NAET® findings again, her eyes suddenly widened and said, "I am so sorry, I forgot about the peanut butter and jelly sandwich I make every morning for my 10-year-old son to take to school for his lunch". Since a peanut butter and jelly sandwich is nutritious and fairly inexpensive and easy to prepare, most parents choose to include the peanut butter sandwiches in their children's school lunches. She did not consider peanut butter in the nut group. She was asked to avoid any contact with the peanut butter for two weeks. She packed a different lunch for her son daily without any trace of nuts or nut oils. Her hand healed nicely in about two weeks. She came in to the office without the gloves. She appeared very happy to go around without gloves. She had not treated for peanuts yet. Just by detecting the allergen and avoiding it her hand healed and the furrows were gone.

Then she was advised to resume making peanut butter sandwiches. If the eczema reappeared, I asked her to return with a sample of the peanut butter so that we could desensitize for the peanut butter. On the following Tuesday (six days later) she returned, both her palms filled with eczema. She said the first two days she did fine. She had some occasional itching in the morning soon after she made the sandwich, but later in the day she felt fine. However on the third day her itching began to get worse. The eczema peaked on Friday, then over the weekend she felt better again. But the exposures on Monday and Tuesday made her return to where she was when she visited my office on the very first day. She had the sample with her. She was treated for the peanut butter immediately and advised to avoid it for 72 hours. She was advised to self-balance her acupressure points every two hours while awake. When she returned after 72 hours, her hands were 90% healed. New baby-like skin was replacing the old diseased skin on the palms of her hands. She was also found to be allergic to all other nuts, hence her aversion for nuts. Her hand eczema completely cleared when she completed the treatments for nuts and a few combination treatments with nuts.

NAET® Specialist Mala Moosad, R.N., L.Ac., N.D., Ph.D., from Buena Park, California, U.S.A., shared this story of a patient with severe foot eczema (allergic contact dermatitis). *A 66-year-old female was seen in our clinic with weeping bilateral foot ulcers* (Figure 2-5). *At the time of arrival in the office she was wearing a pair of rubber slippers. She was walking very slowly, taking each step with extreme caution. She was holding on to her husband's arm for support while walking. She appeared to be in pain. Her major complaint was the chronic eczema on both of her feet, often very painful and weeping without responding to any medication or therapy, for six years. According to her history, the skin on both feet became suddenly extremely itchy and inflamed, causing redness, swelling, cracking, weeping, crusting, and scaling cycle*

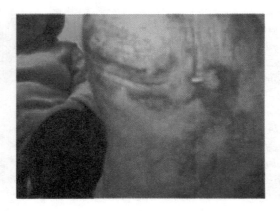

Figure 2-5. Severe foot eczema before NAET® treatment.

since October 2001, after the September 11th incident, for no apparent reason. She tried various topical and oral medications including several courses of cortisone during the six-year period, yet her condition continued to get worse making living impossible. She also suffered from occasional asthma, severe insomnia, constant pain in the knees, feet, anger, and depression, along with a few other symptoms on and off.

Through NAET® testing procedures, the cause of her foot eczema was traced to the rubber footwear that she was wearing. This pair of slippers was weak at all three levels, more so on the emotional level. She was also screened for the NAET® Basic allergens, and she was found to be weak on a physiologic level on all of them. She was also weak on cellular level on most of them. She was also found to be severely allergic to latex, plastics, leather, and synthetic fabrics. When questioned, she told me that she began wearing the rubber slippers in and outside the house since the first sign of eczema in 2001 (six years ago), since they were easy to slip on and take off. Even though the cause of her eczema was pointed towards the latex and rubber allergy, her body did not permit the NAET® on the rubber slippers immediately. Her body desired to go through a series of NAET® Basic allergen treatments before eliminating the sensitivity to the slippers.

The first treatment was brain-body balance formula (BBF). BBF also brought out a strong cellular memory imbalance (hidden emotional trauma from childhood) to the surface-fear, which had six different attachments to it:

- Fear to move forward
- Fear of failure
- Feet freezing due to fear
- Fear of future
- Fear of poverty in the future
- Fear of becoming poor and sick in her old age

78 Freedom From Eczema

Each one had to be addressed alone, and be eliminated one by one, before she cleared the BBF.

That night she slept through the lung and large intestine meridian time (3:00 to 7:00 a.m.) for the first time in six years. Previously, she would wake up coughing, wheezing, and itching between 3:00 to 4:00 a.m., and continue to itch through early morning hours leaving her feet raw, bleeding, and painful.

BBF treatment was followed by the NAET® Basic allergen treatments. Each Basic allergen treatment surfaced a hidden cellular memory imbalance. After each basic treatment, she reported some improvements in different aspects of her health. She felt less anxiety after calcium treatment. The weeping of the foot ulcers reduced after the vitamin C treatment. She was less depressed after the B-complex treatment. Her abnormal sugar craving subsided after sugar treatment. She had cut down on the pain medication by then. The treatments for salt and mineral mix gave her more energy. She continued to itch and bleed through all of these treatments, but with less intensity (Figure 2-6). Her itching reduced greatly after the treatment for grain mix. Even though she made tremendous progress by this point, her foot ulcers were still wet and oozing. The weeping of the wounds was reduced by 50% when she completed the treatment for yeast mix. She improved further when she completed the treatments for stomach acids and base. Then she was also treated for hormones. At this time her body permitted the treatment for the rubber slippers. It took four NAET® sessions to complete treatment on slippers alone. She had collected about 40 pairs of shoes and slippers from various cities and countries — including Spain, France, Mexico, China, etc. — since she thought the problem was due to an allergy to the material that was used in making the shoe or slipper. She was not aware that the emotion connected with the shoe was causing the foot eczema. On September 11, 2001, she had been visiting New York and lived in a hotel in Manhattan, near the twin towers. Hotel guests were evacuated to a safer area and she could not find her shoes or slip-

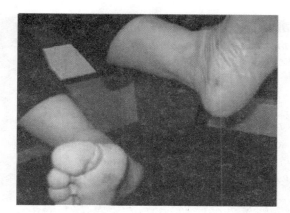

Figure 2-6. Severe foot eczema after 10 NAET® treatments.

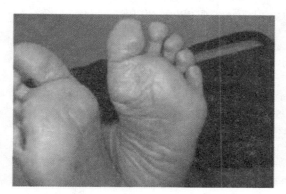

Figure 2-7. Severe foot eczema after 20 NAET® treatments.

pers due to all of the confusion. She found the bathroom slippers and ran out of the area wearing the bathroom slippers. She was confused and scared, not knowing what was going to happen to her. She also had several millions of dollars invested in the twin towers, and lost her entire financial investment. Her future was hopeless and frightening, and her whole body temporarily froze in fear, unable to function or think. After a while she relaxed slightly, but both of her feet remain frozen, unable to even walk a few steps. When she returned to California after a couple of days, she was angry, depressed, sick, and fearful. Soon the eczema started on her feet.

She was initially found to be allergic to all footwear. She was treated four times for different footwear, each one with many cellular memory imbalances. When she completed treatments for four different pairs of slippers, the skin on her feet stopped itching, cracking, bleeding, and weeping (Figure 2-7). *After passing the above four pairs of footwear, she was then retested for all others found previously weak, the untreated 40 pairs of shoes and slippers, and they were all found to be okay. During the course of NAET® treatments, which was three times a week for 12 weeks, she also lost 18 pounds.*

She progressed nicely through the rest of the NAET® Basics. Even though she resolved her original problem, she decided to continue through rest of the NAET® Classic allergens to prevent possible recurrences of the same or similar problems in the future. In addition, she was treated with NAET® for all of her other known sensitivities, intolerances, and allergies, which revealed numerous cellular memory imbalances that had accumulated since childhood. All of these cellular memory imbalances were causing obstacles in her healing. They were the roadblocks that prevented her from responding to medications and therapies during the past six years. When she completed treatment for 40 NAET® Classic allergens at all three levels of healing, she began to feel lie herself again. Finally, eczema was no longer a problem. She no longer needed to take any medications (topical ointments and pain medications).

One year after completing her NAET® treatments, she still remains free of her eczema.

Irritant Contact Dermatitis

This is a type of eczema caused by frequent contact with everyday substances, such as detergents and chemicals, which are irritating to the skin. It most commonly occurs on the hands of adults and can be prevented by avoiding the irritants and keeping the skin moisturized. About 75% of contact dermatitis cases are of the irritant type, which is the most common occupational skin disease. Irritant eczema can occur by contacting or being near corrosive chemicals and the reaction can often be instant as in contact with poison ivy, paint thinner, wet paint, wood varnish, tile and floor cleaning liquid chemicals, automobile cleaning or polishing agents, etc.

A Sampling of Contactant Allergies

Allergy to Fabrics

People can be allergic to the clothes they wear daily, which can cause eczema. Patients can be allergic to synthetic fabrics, such as nylon, or even natural fabrics, such as cotton or wool. For example, some people cannot wear wool without breaking out in rashes. Some people who are sensitive to wool also react to creams with a lanolin base, since lanolin is derived from sheep's wool. Some people can be allergic to socks made of cotton, Orlon®, wool, and develop symptoms of knee pain, etc. People can also be allergic to carpets and drapes, causing eczema on the feet or ankles.

Allergy to Yeast and *Candida*

Persistent yeast infections are frequently seen in females. Some female patients are allergic to their pantyhose and suffer from leg cramps, high blood pressure, swollen legs, psoriasis, and persistent yeast infections. Toilet paper, cornstarch, corn products, and paper towels also cause problems that mimic yeast infections in many people.

Allergy to Cosmetics

Many people are allergic to makeup products, lipsticks, face creams, skin lotions, underarm deodorants and antiperspirants. These allergies can cause skin rashes, irritation of the skin, dermatitis, boils, infections, lymph gland swelling, and pain. The chemicals in antiperspirants and deodorants are toxic, causing eczema and other skin problems in sensitive individuals.

In one of my patients, the use of a popular skin cream was the cause of the beginning of skin cancer. She was allergic to vitamin A and to the skin cream itself. After she was treated with NAET® for these substances, her lesions cleared up.

Allergy to Sunscreens

Some people find that sunscreens can make their eczema worse. It is important to always be careful, testing a small amount of any new sunscreen on a small part of the body, before applying it to the whole body.

Allergy to Heavy Metals

Heavy metal toxicity is on the rise. Most foods are sprayed with pesticides. Pesticides are loaded with heavy metals such as mercury. Mercury is a neurotoxin that is used in most pesticides to help immobilize the pests. Mercury is a neurotoxin for humans too. People can be exposed to mercury from dental fillings, childhood immunizations, fish, and pesticides. Pressed wood, decorative woodwork, and some furniture items are treated with pesticide derivatives to increase longevity.

Allergy to Jewelry

People can be allergic to the jewelry they wear, and sometimes to the jewelry that others wear. They may also be allergic to such items when visiting friends, shopping, attending theaters, or going anywhere that people congregate. These allergies can cause eczema.

For 10 years, a young man had constant yeast infections, chronic fatigue syndrome, emotional fatigue, night sweats, nervousness, poor memory, and various mental disturbances. He had seen a number of medical doctors, chiropractors, acupuncturists, and nutritionists to get some relief. Often suicidal, he was going for psychiatric counseling regularly. He was treated in our office for various allergies for over six months and showed marked progress.

He stopped having night sweats and fatigue, his memory improved, and the yeast infection cleared up for the first time in 10 years. He began to live normally once again. He was very happy and had a new girlfriend for a few months, when all of a sudden he returned to our office in tears. He said he was almost back to where he had started. We tested him for the various items that he was once treated for and found no allergy to anything. We noticed that he was wearing a lot of jewelry: four earrings, with four different stones in one ear, a heavy necklace with a huge gold and silver pendant, eight rings on the fingers with stones (including star ruby, diamond, emerald, garnet, turquoise, and sapphire) and a gold watch studded with diamonds. When he was tested for the stones, he was found to be highly allergic to them. He revealed that he had taken off all the jewelry when he was treated for minerals in our office and did not put them back until recently. He was fond of jewelry and for 10 years had always adorned himself with these jewels. Since he was feeling better, he started wearing them again and all the previous symptoms returned. He was treated for all the jewelry and once again he became healthy and happy. Moderation is the one word that can keep everyone out of agony.

Allergy to Crystals and Stones

Most often, wearing crystals and stones can lead to stiffness, pain in the shoulders and upper back, tension, itching, hives, eczema, or acne. Some people decorate their office desks with crystals and stones, while others use writing pens and clip boards studded with crystals or stones. Constant contact with crystals and stones can cause skin irritation and eczema in such people, though they probably never suspect these precious stones or crystal as the culprits.

One of my patients, a doctor who had a passion for crystals, decorated his office table with crystals of different sizes that touched against his forearms while he was working at his desk. There was a crystal holder for his pen, and several crystals stuck on the clipboard that he used often. He suffered from chronic itching and eczema on his forearm, and his condition did not respond to any medication. He was advised to remove all of the crystals from his desk for a couple of weeks. By then his itching stopped and his eczema cleared up. He was asked to bring all of the crystals to his desk again. Within hours, all of his itching (and the skin irritation due to that itching) returned. Then he was treated with NAET® and advised to avoid all the crystals for a week. The NAET® testing indicated that he needed to avoid the crystals for a week instead of the usual 25 hours because he had a severe allergy to crystals. On the following week his skin was normal without any irritation or itching, and he was no longer bothered by the crystals on his desk.

Allergy to Crude Oil

Many people are allergic to crude oils and their derivatives, which include plastics, synthetic rubber products, telephones, the naugahyde-covered chairs, milk containers, polyester fabrics, and face/body creams. Crude oil products cause skin irritation in sensitive individuals.

Allergy to Formaldehyde and Building Materials

Formaldehyde is found in fabrics, newspaper, ink, pressed wood, sheet rock, building materials, new carpet, name tags on clothes, paints, etc. Many people have been diagnosed as suffering from "sick-building syndrome". People who work in the newspaper industry, including writers, can suffer from eczema, itching, hives, or carpal tunnel syndrome, which can often be from an allergy to formaldehyde or plastic.

Allergy to Latex

To most people, latex gloves can be very helpful items, but to many people, latex gloves are allergens. Latex gloves are one of the most common items found in hospitals, and hardly any procedure is done in the hospitals without them. Dentists, cosmetologists, and other health professionals also use latex gloves for their procedures. Unfortunately, latex gloves can cause severe hand eczema. If this condition is not taken care of immediately, it may even spread to other areas of the body.

A 48-year-old woman went to the dentist for a routine cleaning. The dental hygienist put on a pair of latex gloves and began cleaning her teeth. All of a sudden, her body became burning hot. The patient almost went into anaphylactic shock. The doctor came in and called the paramedics who revived her with the help of drugs. She had red rashes all over her body and a mild fever when she left the dentist's office. She came to our office two days later with red rashes still on her body and a fever of 100 degrees Fahrenheit.

NAET® testing showed that she was allergic to the latex gloves used by the dental hygienist. She was also allergic to the chalk powder in the gloves, which affected her large intestine, heart, and gallbladder meridians. She was treated for the gloves and the powder. After she was treated for the gloves, she was also treated for local anesthetics, amalgam, cleaning agents, gauze, and cotton balls. She was advised to return to the dental office to finish up the dental work. This time, she had no adverse reaction. She even had a root canal procedure. Later, she revealed that the allergy elimination treatment for latex gloves and powder was the best thing that had happened to her in 15 years. She had been afraid to have any intimate relationship with her husband for many years. She reacted to his semen and broke out in rashes and blisters all over her body whenever they had intercourse. Actually, she was allergic to the condom materials and could not use them or be around them. Later, she was successfully treated for her husband's semen, and it goes without saying that she is now a very happy woman.

Other Career-Produced Allergies

Many common allergies that cause skin problems are related to a person's job. For example: cooks (spices, cooking oil smells), waiters (smell of the foods, plastic trays), grocery store employees (various items ranging from chemicals to the fresh food found in the store), clerks (paper products, inks, liquid paper, permanent markers), gardeners (pesticides, herbicides, plants, tools, leaf-blowers), computer programmers (computer radiation, plastics, electrical cords, mouse, keyboard, monitor), teachers (white board, chalk, pens, markers, paper, glue), bakers (flour, eggs, baking powder, artificial colors, flavorings, food chemicals), surgeons (latex gloves, gowns, masks, surgical instruments, antiseptics), and lawyers (paper, pens, markers, computers, books, leather chair, wooden office furniture, cell phones). Virtually no trade or skill is exempt from being exposed to allergens that can trigger eczema.

Skin Conditions Associated With Contact Allergens

Though it is tempting to write about one symptom for each common allergen, it would make this book much too long. However, it might reveal how contactants (which could also include contact with ingestants, inhalants, etc.) can affect people to produce symptoms often diagnosed as "incurable", such as when doctors tell patients, "learn to live with it". Many people spend their entire life visiting doctors and taking medications, still not finding any relief from their suffering. This author was one of them, before discovering NAET®. When a person learns to identify the cause of the problem, at least that cause can be avoided, which in itself will produce some relief. Perhaps the following list of some common problems (with the associated allergen in brackets), which were identified and relieved with NAET®, may assist readers to search for culprits that just might be seemingly innocent daily contactants.

- Acne on the arms and legs (razor blade)
- Acne on the baby (cotton clothes)
- Acne and stiff neck (jewelry, high-neck fabrics)
- Acne and vulvodynea (fabrics, oxalic acids, berries)
- Acne on the back (fried foods)
- Acne on the front and back of the trunk (body lotion)
- Acne rosacea (fruits, sugar)
- Athlete's foot (shoes, socks)
- Baldness, hair loss (cotton towel for the head; Vitamin C, A, iron)
- Blepharitis (eye brow pencil)
- Blisters on the lips (computer keyboard)
- Boils on the inguinal area and vulva (elastic)
- Boils all over the body (gelatin)
- Boils and carbuncles on the body (jogging suit, fleece)
- Candidiasis under breast (bra)
- Cellulitis (dry cleaning chemical)
- Chloracne (swimming pool water)
- Chronic dermatitis of the hands and feet (milk)
- Contact dermatitis (table rose)
- Cracked nipples (baby's saliva)
- Cradle cap (breast milk)
- Dandruff (new shampoo)
- Dermatitis on the face (liquid make-up)
- Diaper rash (city tap water; diapers, vitamin A & D cream; soy based Formula)
- Dry skin on the upper body and both feet (cotton shirt, cotton socks)
- Dry skin, peeling skin (talcum powder)
- Dryness and itching below the knees (elastic, nylons)
- Eczema – Stasis (ankle jewelry, cotton socks)
- Eczema – weeping on the groin and vulva (candidiasis, staphylococcus)
- Eczema – wet around navel (jewelry: navel ring)
- Eczema (polyester shirt)
- Eczema around groin, around rectum, upper thigh (cotton underwear, toilet tissue)
- Eczema on a baby (baby lotion)
- Eczema on feet (fabric: bedroom slippers)
- Eczema on hand, plus dry skin (newspaper)

- Eczema on hand, plus tennis elbow (computer mouse)
- Eczema on hands for five years in a pediatric nurse (latex gloves)
- Eczema on the lower back (elastic)
- Eczema on the mid-back (elastic, metal)
- Eczema on the neck (name tag on the shirt)
- Eczema on the whole body (saliva)
- Eczema on the wrist and finger joints (table tennis racket)
- Eczema, vulvodynea (wood furniture, body lotion with vitamin C products)
- Fungus on the toes (grains)
- Genital warts (elastics, cotton crotch, toilet seat)
- Hair loss in female (birth control pill; hair brush)
- Hives (humidity, dampness; reading newspaper; upholstery, fabric, dust, animals)
- Hives on the baby (bathing water)
- Hives, abdominal cramps (newspaper)
- Hives, heat rash, warm body (humidity)
- Hives, sneezing attacks (smell from flowers, perfumes; smell from frying chicken)
- Hives, swelling on the face (grass, pollen)
- Itching (fabrics, jewelry)
- Itching all over the body (rayon fabrics)
- Itching and joint pains (weather change, fabrics)
- Itching and tennis elbow (tennis racket, ball, glove)
- Itching and vulvodynea (underwear, elastics)
- Itching on the face, neck (down pillow)
- Itching on the legs below knee (woolen socks)
- Itching on the neck and back (jewelry)
- Itching on the right thigh (television remote control)
- Jock itch (cotton underwear; elastics on the underpants and pants)
- Leathery skin (sweat suit)
- Lice infection (louse)
- Miliary rash on the baby (body lotion)
- *Molluscum contagiosum* (soy milk)
- Paget's disease of the nipple (bra)
- Peeling skin on the lower abdomen (bathing suit)
- Perioral dermatitis (tooth brush, city water)
- Photosensitivity (sun, Vitamin D, magnesium)
- Psoriasis (milk products; saliva; spices)
- Psoriasis of the mid back (elastic, cottage cheese)
- Rashes (parasites; sun, heat, fabrics, water)
- Rashes all over the body, especially on the trunk (dry cleaned blouse)
- Rashes and hives (tap water, bathing water)
- Rashes and stomach aches (cooking, touching food products during preparation)
- Rashes on the face and exposed area of the skin (smell of seasoning spice)
- Raynaud's disease (silk)
- Ringworm (knee highs, socks, pants)
- Scabies (fabrics)
- Scaly skin on the legs (fabric, socks, shoe)
- Scleroderma (milk, egg, sugar)

- Skin cancer (razor blade; sun radiation)
- Skin tags (gold jewelry)
- Spider veins (stockings, fluffy bathroom slippers)
- Swelling of the body (water, cold)
- Swelling on the face (wood smoke, barbeque sauce)
- Ulcers on the sole of the foot (bathroom slippers)
- Ulcers (weeping) around the waist (fabrics, elastics)
- Uterine fibroid (cotton fabrics)

INJECTANTS

Injectants are allergens that are inserted into the body through the skin, muscles, joints, or blood vessels in the form of various serums, antitoxins, vaccines, and drugs.

Allergy to Insect Bites and Stings

Many people react to bites from insects. Spider and flea bites can be fatal in some cases. Many people react to wasp and bee stings. One NAET® Specialist shared this story: *A patient came in with many painful spider bites on her swollen arms after working in her vegetable garden. The next time she came in to see me, she brought a dead spider from the garden. I treated her with NAET® for allergy to the spider. After treatment, her wounds healed, and she was no longer bothered by spider bites from her garden.*

Allergy to Injectable Drugs

Allergy to such injectables as vaccination, immunization (e.g., diptheria/polio/tetanus [DPT], measles/mumps/rubella [MMR], Hepatitis B), insulin, allergy shots, and other injectable drugs can trigger eczema. For example: *One patient's whole left hand eczema started after she received a BCG vaccination 10 years ago in India. When she was desensitized with NAET® for BCG, her 10-year-old itching and eczema conditions cleared.*

Individuals with eczema are at special risk for developing extensive vaccine-related lesions, through direct inoculation of the virus onto diseased skin. A rare but severe adverse reaction to smallpox vaccination is called eczema vaccinatum; if smallpox is not an immediate risk, this vaccination should not be given to persons with eczema or atopic dermatitis.

Eczema herpeticum is caused by allergy to chicken pox vaccination or herpes zoster or simplex virus (HSV), and occurs mainly in people with atopic dermatitis. Secondary bacterial skin infections may be one of the causes for this type of infection. The most common bacteria affecting the condition may be *Streptococcus aureus,* group A-hemolytic *Streptococcus,* and *Pseudomonas.*

In Case of Emergency

Most NAET® patients become well prepared to take care of their own unexpected emergencies if they encounter any situations when they are traveling. By the time they complete their NAET® Basic allergen treatments, their NAET® Specialist will teach them self-balancing techniques (see Chapter 4). However, patients with acute symptoms should also seek qualified emergency assistance when needed.

INFECTANTS

Infectants are allergens that produce their effect by causing a sensitivity to an infectious agent, such as bacteria, virus, or parasite. It should be noted that infectious agents are contacted in many ways. Casual contact with objects and people exposes a person daily to dangerous contaminants and possible illnesses. When the person's autoimmune system is functioning properly, that person can pass off the illness without notice. However, when the person's autoimmune system is not working at maximum performance levels, then infections, fevers, etc. can result. For example: *Maxine, a 72-year-old woman, had chronic weeping ulcers on the tips of the fingers of both her hands for many years, and had tried all possible medicines and ointments. Her medical history revealed that caring for roses was her main hobby. She was tested for roses by neuromuscular sensitivity testing (NST) and was found to be highly allergic to them. When she was treated with NAET® for roses, her chronic ulcers healed nicely.*

Autosensitization (Autoeczematization)

Autoeczematization (the spread of eczema lesions from an original focused skin area) is a reaction to infection with parasites, fungi, bacteria, viruses, yeast, *Candida*, or mold. The appearance of the skin response varies depending on the cause. The eczema always occurs some distance away from the original infection. It is completely curable with the clearance of the original infection.

Diaper Rash

Diaper rash is an inflammatory reaction localized to the skin area usually covered by the diaper. It can have many causes, including infections (yeast, bacterial, or viral), friction irritation, chemical allergies (perfumes, soaps), sweat, or plugged sweat glands.

Head Lice

This problem is very common among school children. Head lice are small greyish parasitic insects that live only on human scalps. They cannot fly, jump, or burrow into the scalp, but their six legs are perfectly adapted for clinging firmly onto scalp hairs. Their presence imply that the person is allergic to them, and does not imply a lack of cleanliness. After treated with NAET® for lice allergy, these parasites may leave the body silently since they find the body no longer to be an ideal home.

Scabies

Scabies is a common and very itchy skin condition caused by human scabies mites. The mites that cause scabies are tiny eight-legged parasites, smaller than a pinhead. They usually find their way from one person to another through prolonged direct skin-to-skin contact with someone who already has scabies. These mites only rarely find their way to a person from objects such as clothing or bedding. As with head lice, the presence of scabies mites implies that the person is allergic to them, and after the allergies are desensitized with NAET®, the scabies mites may leave the body silently since they find the body no longer to be an ideal home.

PHYSICAL AGENTS

Physical agents include cold, heat, sunlight, dampness, dryness, humidity, drafts, fog, smog, mechanical irritants (such as vibration or sound), or electromagnetic energy. Physical agents that cause allergic reactions and skin reactions are called physical allergens. Patients suffering from more than one allergy can be deeply affected by physical allergens.

Allergy to Cold

A patient who has already eaten some allergic foods, then walks in cold air or drafts, might develop upper respiratory problems, sore throat, asthma, itching, hives, or eczema, depending on that patient's tendency toward health-related problems. Some people are very sensitive to cold or heat, and produce itching and eczema whether or not they have eaten any allergic food. Such cases are common.

As with other types of allergic responses, physical allergy to cold may be manifested as:

- Hives or angioneurotic edema (swelling caused by dilation of capillaries) of the hands when washed in cold water, and hives on areas of the body exposed to cold air
- Swelling of the lips or spasms of the stomach after eating cold foods
- Allergic rhinitis and asthma after inhalation of cold air (responds well to the NAET® wind and dampness treatment)
- Skin turning blue in cold air and red under a warm sun

Low concentrations of certain nutrients can throw the body into imbalance and extreme discomfort when the weather changes. Lack of iron, Vitamin B12, and folic acid may cause poor blood quality and inadequate circulation, blocking the body's ability to exchange oxygen and carbon dioxide properly, then adding more difficulties in extreme temperatures. Many patients who have extremely cold feet or cold hands suffer from poor circulation.

Allergy to Heat

Some people are very sensitive to hot weather or heat, and exposure to heat can produce itching, hives, or eczema. Heat rash is a skin irritation caused by excessive sweating during hot, humid weather. It can occur at any age but is most common in young children. Heat rash looks like a red cluster of pimples or small blisters. It is more likely to occur on the neck and upper chest, in the groin, under the breasts, and in elbow creases.

A patient suffered from hives, itching, and redness of the skin, headache, diarrhea, general weakness, and fainting spells whenever she walked in the hot sun, drank hot liquids, or took a hot or warm shower. She was treated with NAET® for hot water, and has not reacted nearly as much to heat since.

A 38-year-old woman had second-degree burns with huge blisters as a result of a container of boiling water falling on her. After one week of extreme pain, she was treated with NAET® for very hot water in a glass jar. After 24 hours the pain was gone. Within a week, her skin was healed.

Photodermatitis

Heat rash and itchy spots can be caused by sensitivity to sunlight. Many people find that their eczema improves with exposure to sunlight (this is particularly true of the contact and discoid types) while others experience a worsening of their condition. In either case, the skin will still need protection from the sun's rays in the summer.

One of the young patients who came to our office had a history of canker sores whenever he walked in the sun. He was highly allergic to Vitamin D, one of the vitamins produced in the body with the help of sunlight. After he was treated with NAET® for Vitamin D, the incidents of canker sores as a result of walking in the sun diminished.

Exercise-Induced Eczema

It is very important for the body to maintain proper circulation of blood and nutrients to the vital organs and to each and every cell in the body. Proper blood circulation is also important to eliminate toxins from the body. Healthy adrenal glands hold the key to better health by maintaining a healthy immune system. Someone with a good immune system will manifest fewer allergies and skin reactions. Exercise-induced eczema has been seen more frequently since fitness programs have become more popular around the country. Endorphins and enkephalins are produced in large amounts during exercise. These are the brain enzymes that produce a sense of well-being. It is possible for patients to be allergic to their own endorphins and other hormones, which cause itching and skin problems. These patients should first be treated with NAET® for endorphins and other specific hormones before they begin a vigorous exercise program.

Allergy to People or Pets

When a patient comes close to the energy field of another person, or a pet, if that other energy field happens to be incompatible with the patient, then a repulsion of the two energy fields takes place. The other person (or pet) that is capable of producing the repulsion between those energy fields is considered an allergen to the patient.

Eczema can be due to an allergy to people. The patient may be allergic to a caretaker, parent, sibling, spouse, therapist, school classmate, teacher, student, etc.

Some people consider their pet as a family member; for some people, their pet may be their only family. Unfortunately many people have an allergy to pets, either through contact with hair and dander, or due to the pet's electromagnetic energy field. Pet allergy can trigger skin disorders, including hives, eczema, and itching.

GENETIC CAUSES

One path to achieving optimum health is the discovery of possible tendencies toward allergies inherited from parents and grandparents. Allergies can also skip generations and be manifested very differently in children. Many people with various allergic manifestations respond well to treatment for the various disease agents that have been transmitted from parents. Many skin disorders, both common and rare, are being linked to genes.

Some studies have found psoriasis to be as much as 90% genetic and 10% environmental. Studies reported in the July 2005 issue of the *Journal of the American Academy of Dermatology* suggest that in twins, there is a 67% chance of developing psoriasis if an identical twin has psoriasis, but only a 18% chance of developing psoriasis if a nonidentical (fraternal) twin has psoriasis. Researchers are trying to determine which genes may play a role in this autoimmune disease. Many of these genes seem to be located on the short arm of chromosome 6, an area responsible for immune responses in the body.

Researchers have found that rare skin disorders, such as ichthyosis (dry rectangular scales on the skin, resembling fish scales), are inherited disorders caused by specific defective genes. Gene mutations for this disorder seem to be located on chromosome 1.

Atopic Eczema

Atopic eczema (also called infantile eczema, flexural eczema, or atopic dermatitis) is believed to have a genetic component, and often runs in families. Atopic eczema is the most common form of eczema and is closely linked with asthma and hay fever. It can affect both children and adults. One of the most common symptoms of atopic eczema is itchiness (or pruritus), which can be almost unbearable. The itchy rash is particularly noticeable on the face and scalp, neck, the inside of the elbows, behind the knees, and on the buttocks. Other symptoms include overall dryness of the skin, redness, and inflammation. Constant scratching can also cause the skin to split, leaving it prone to infection. In infected eczema the skin may crack and ooze (wet eczema).

The exact cause of atopic eczema/dermatitis is unknown, but a genetic predisposition may be aggravated by such factors as food allergies, infections, irritating chemicals, temperature, humidity, and emotions. Approximately 10% of childhood cases are due to allergy to certain foods, particularly eggs, peanuts, milk, fish, soy, and wheat. Atopic dermatitis tends to flare up in response to extremes in temperature and humidity. Other causes of flare-ups are sweating and psychological stress.

Atopic eczema/dermatitis is most commonly seen in infants, usually developing between the age of one month and one year, commonly in those with strong family histories of atopic disease. At least half of those cases clear by age 36 months. These children often acquire other atopic disorders as they grow older. Typically, this form of dermatitis flares and subsides repeatedly before finally resolving during adolescence. However, it can persist into adulthood. In adults, atopic eczema is generally chronic or recurring.

Mark, age 28, suffered from eczema and severe acne on his face, back, and upper neck. He showed the need to treat for bacteria mix. After treatment with NAET® for the bacteria, he responded nicely, with most of the acne clearing on his back. However some of the acne and eczema remained on his face. Upon questioning him, it was found that his mother suffered from scarlet fever as a child. He was immediately tested and treated with NAET® for Streptococcus *mix. His remaining eczema and acne cleared up nicely when he successfully completed NAET® treatment for* Streptococcus *group.*

MOLDS AND FUNGI

Molds and fungi are in a category by themselves, because of the numerous ways they are contacted as allergens in everyday life. They can be ingested, inhaled, touched, or even (as with penicillin) injected. They come in many forms: airborne spores, making up a large part of the dust people breathe or pick up in vacuum cleaners; fluids such as drinking water; dark fungal growth in the corners of damp rooms; athlete's foot; and, in particularly obnoxious vaginal conditions commonly called "yeast infections". They grow on trees and in the damp soil. They are a source of food, as in truffles and mushrooms; of diseases such as ringworm and the aforementioned yeast infections; and of healing, as in the tremendous benefits mankind has derived from the drug penicillin.

Athlete's foot is a human parasitic fungus that grows anywhere in the body, where the area is fairly moist and not exposed to sunlight or air. It is particularly difficult to eliminate, and treatment generally consists of a topical preparation, multiple daily cleansing of the area, a medicinal powder, and wearing light cotton socks to avoid further infection from dyes used in colored apparel. Allergies to cotton, Orlon®, nylon, or paper could result in the explosions of infections including ascomycetes fungi (yeast) that women are finding so troublesome. Feminine tampons, toilet papers, douches, and deodorants can also cause yeast infections.

Waterbeds are comfortable places for molds to grow when the user forgets to add chemicals regularly into the water inside to inhibit growth of molds. Users must also be careful to test the chemicals for possible allergic reactions. When sleeping in untreated waterbeds, many chronic problems can develop, including chronic bronchitis in spite of taking repeated antibiotics, chronic sinusitis, migraines, back aches, itching, and skin rashes.

PSYCHOGENIC CAUSES

Many times, the origin of physical symptoms can be traced back to some unresolved emotional trauma. At the cellular level, each cell in the body has the capability to respond physically, physiologically and psychologically to our daily activities. When the vital energy flows evenly and uninterrupted through the energy pathways (acupuncture meridians), the body functions normally. When there is a disruption (an increase or decrease) in the energy flow through the meridians, energy blockages can occur, causing various emotional symptoms in those particular meridians. According to Oriental medical theory, there are seven major emotions which can cause pathological health problems in people: sadness affects lung meridian, joy affects the heart meridian, disgust affects the stomach meridian, anger affects the liver meridian, worry affects the spleen meridian, fear affects the kidney meridian, and depression affects the pericardium meridian. Further information on meridians and emotional connections is available in Chapter 10 of *Say Good-bye to Illness* (see this author's listings in the bibliography section at the end of this book).

People with skin disorders have delicate emotions. Any simple emotional incident can sometimes imprint a lasting image in their minds causing itching and scratching. This author has treated hundreds of patients with eczema, and 90% of them have had an emotionally traumatic past. In most cases, some traumatic emotional event from the past may have triggered the itching and skin problems. Probably the brain used this defense mechanism in order to protect the body, but after the need was completed, the brain could not return to its original state. Addressing the exact issue from the past that had triggered the signal to react adversely, using NAET® to help balance the emotional status, helps to stop the exaggerated reactions to the environment so that people can resume normal life.

Martha suffered from whole-body, weeping eczema since the age of 21. She was 48 when her parents brought her for NAET® treatments. Martha said she began having eczema rather suddenly when she turned 21. Everything in her foods, drinks, and environment triggered severe uncontrollable itching and eczema. She was started on NAET® Basic allergen treatments. Several emotions, suchc as inferiority complex, low self-esteem, depression, etc., were treated during this process. Then came we discovered that she was highly allergic to ocean water. A fear for ocean water showed up on the testing. The date of the fear causing the emotional trauma was her 21st birthday. After searching through her memory with her parents' help, she remembered that they had gone to San Francisco to celebrate her 21st birthday. While she was walking at the pier, she happened to see a man entertaining the public by singing and playing drums. He had no legs. Both of his legs were cut off at the hip. But he was sitting on a wooden board and showing different tricks by spinning a wooden board around and dragging it across with his hip, etc. He also had an associate with him, who had only one leg. Martha felt sorry for them, so she moved closer to the man with one leg and asked him how they lost their legs. He said they were war veterans, and the legs were lost fighting in a war.

Suddenly she felt like fainting. Her father was standing next to her listening to their conversation. He watched her face become pale while talking to him, then saw her passing out, so he held her in his arms in a split second to prevent her from falling down. He laid her on a nearby bench and sprinkled some water on her face. They returned to their hotel immediately. She became very sick the next day, with nausea and internal tremors. She recovered after resting for a week. She had just finished her schooling, and after vacation she was going to look for a job. She was also engaged to a young man who had gone to serve in the army four years ago.

He was coming home to see her and possibly to marry her during his next vacation, which would be in about two months. By the time she recovered from her last episode, she received a letter from her fiancé saying that he would be on vacation one month earlier than he had anticipated. He was coming home the following week and he wanted to marry her then.

That night she started itching all over her body and she could not sleep. By the next morning, her whole body was swollen and bleeding in many places. She still continued to itch nonstop. She was taken to the family doctor, then later to a dermatologist, but none of the treatments gave her any relief.

On the following week when her fiancé came to see her she was in a very pathetic condition. He tried to talk to her and he wanted to be near her but she refused to see him in this shape and asked him to break the engagement. She refused to marry him. He returned to army service without marriage. She continued to be sick. The following year when he came on vacation, she insisted that he marry someone else. She totally refused to even talk to him. Finally he found someone else and got married and moved away from her hometown.

She continued to stay in bed, itching and scratching, and remained in full disability for all of those years. She consulted with every specialist and tried every possible therapy and treatment, but she reacted adversely to all treatments. Then someone told her about NAET® and she came to our office for treatment.

We discovered this story through NAET® diagnostic methods: She became frightened when she saw those war veterans without limbs. Her subconscious mind warned her that her fiancé was in the service; she feared that he might return home to her without legs, and that she would then have to live with the man without legs. That thought frightened her, and her body reacted by itching, scratching, and producing whole-body weeping eczema. If her body became disfigured with weeping eczema her fiancé would leave her alone. Her subconscious mind decided that she would rather live alone than go through the pain and agony of watching a limbless man living with her for the rest of her life.

So, she was treated with NAET® for that fear. She had to be treated four times just to clear that fear about the whole event. Her eczema cleared nicely: about 90% was gone after she completed the treatment for that main fear. She continued to be treated with NAET® for various other fears and emotions that she had collected during the 27 years of her illness. She became normal when she completed her treatments.

The NAET® emotional blockage removal treatment was able to turn off the fear-switch, and the fear that she had towards all military servicemen. Along with that, her brain turned off the switch towards eczema. The human brain is a fascinating instrument with hundreds of hidden secret keys.

Eczema Due to Stress

Eczema can be caused by stress overload, an inability to handle the stress of daily life, insomnia, or other stress-related issues. The mind, body, and spirit are inseparable. Disease therefore is often a result of an imbalance between mind, body, and spirit. If we do not balance our body at all three levels, we cannot achieve complete health.

CHAPTER 3

HOW ARE ALLERGY-RELATED SKIN DISORDERS DIAGNOSED?

Finding the Underlying Problem

OVERVIEW

*A*llergic conditions are more frequently associated with skin disorders, especially eczema, than most people realize. Statistics show that at least 50% of the U.S. population suffers from some form of allergy, and that every year there are more recognized cases of allergy-related skin disorders.

Diagnosis of skin disorders should always include detailed medical history, physical examination, and appropriate laboratory tests if necessary. Because many people are interested in understanding conventional Western medicine and Oriental medicine diagnostic methods, basic information will be included here for general perspective and comparison. However, the purpose of this book is to describe something new: the NAET® diagnostic approach, so more emphasis will be given to this method, with comments regarding how Western, Oriental, and Applied Kinesiological methods are integrated into this unique approach .

WESTERN MEDICINE
DIAGNOSTIC APPROACH

Scratch Test

Western medical allergists generally depend on skin testing (scratch test, patch test, etc.), in which a very small amount of a suspected allergic substance is introduced into the person's skin through a scratch or an injection. The site of injection is observed for any reaction. If there is any reaction at the area of injection, the person is considered to be allergic to that substance. Each item has to be tested individually.

Laboratory Investigations

Complete blood count, blood chemistry and thyroid profile should be done to rule out anemia, infections, thyroid disorders, diabetes, etc.

Special blood tests, called the enzyme-linked immunosorbent assay (ELISA), can determine the level of a patient's environmental allergens, (e.g., house dust mite, cockroaches, indoor plants) to confirm that the patient is atopic (allergic). The ELISA test can also identify specific allergens that are causing symptoms, as well as any cross-reactions to the foods eaten on a daily basis (e.g., patients with latex allergy may also react to avocado, bananas, and chestnuts). This is because there are common or cross-reacting biological elements in these somewhat unrelated foods.

Screening for Atopy

The family history is the most useful predictor of atopy (allergy) in young children. For small children with atopic dermatitis, food allergy screen is extremely useful. This test detects specific IgE to the common foods (e.g., milk, egg, peanut, wheat, fish, soya) which are known to play a role in the disease process.

Total Serum IgE

Total serum IgE is usually very high in children with atopic dermatitis, particularly in those with severe disease. When the total serum IgE is very high, specific IgE radioallergosorbent (RAST) tests may also be elevated.

Allergen-Specific IgE

Allergen-specific IgE is conveniently determined by the ImmunoCAP RAST test, available in 90% of laboratories around the country.

Mixed Allergen Tests

Mixed allergen tests have been developed to enable the practitioner to cost effectively screen for specific IgE to groups of similar allergens, e.g., fish mixes, spice mixes, or grain mixes. If the mixed allergen test is positive, specific ImmnoCAP RAST tests of the component allergens will identify the culprit.

Measuring Eosinophilia

Eosinophilia is a characteristic in patients with allergic skin disease, e.g., eczema or drug-induced urticaria (hives). Eosinophils are a type of white blood cell, and eosinophil counts may decrease as the patients go into remission or are removed from the allergen responsible for their symptoms.

Serum Tryptase

Tryptase is secreted exclusively by mast cells (also called mastocytes, a type of cell that is often injured in allergic reactions). Tryptase is not normally detectable in the serum of healthy or allergic individuals. In situation where there has been massive mast cell activation, e.g., anaphylaxis or mastocytosis, the tryptase level assessment may help with diagnosis.

Microscopic Examination

Microscopic examination involves a scraping or swab of the affected area, which is then sent to the laboratory for examination under a microscope.

Culturing

Culturing involves a sterile swab that is rubbed on the infected or affected skin surface, and sent to the laboratory for controlled growth of the organisms. Evaluation of these samples can help detect and identify infectious processes, or sensitivity to antibiotics.

Elimination Diet

The elimination diet was developed by Albert H. Rowe, M.D. of Oakland, California. This approach consists of a very limited diet that must be followed for a period long enough to determine whether or not any of the foods included in it are responsible for the allergic symptoms. The importance of adhering strictly to the diet during the diagnostic period is very crucial.

ORIENTAL MEDICINE
DIAGNOSTIC APPROACH

An allergy means an altered reactivity. Western medicine uses various standard diagnostic tests to measure reactions and after-effects. Energy medicine has also developed various devices to measure the reactions. Oriental medicine has used *"Medical I Ching"* since 3,322 BC, and this approach is the basis for the simple, kinesiological neuromuscular sensitivity testing (NST) discussed in the NAET® approach later in this chapter. Study of the acupuncture meridians, which are an integral part of Oriental medicine, is helpful to understand NST and how it works.

All living beings have energy meridians and nerve energy circulates through these meridians throughout the day and night (see Figures 3-1 and 3-2). If one learns to identify abnormal symptoms associated with acupuncture meridians, as described on the following pages, detection of the causative agents (allergens) will be easier.

According to Oriental medicine, energy disturbances in the lung and large intestine lead to various types of skin disorders. However, according to NAET® findings, all meridians can be associated with skin problems since they all are interconnected directly or indirectly. Any allergen can cause blockage in one or more of the meridians at the same time. If the allergen is causing blockages in only one meridian, the patient may demonstrate symptoms related to that particular meridian. The intensity of the symptoms will depend on the severity of the blockage. The patient may suffer from one symptom, many symptoms or all the symptoms of this blocked meridian. Sometimes a patient can have many meridians blocked at the same time. In such cases, the patient may demonstrate a variety of symptoms, one symptom from each meridian, or many symptoms from certain meridians and one or two

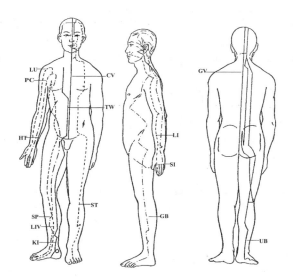

Figure 3-1.
Energy flow
through 12
meridians.

CV = Conception Vessel meridian; GB = Gall Bladder meridian; GV = Governing Vessel meridian; Ht = Heart meridian; Kid = Kidney meridian; LI = Large Intestine meridian; Liv = Liver meridian; Lu = Lung meridian; Pc = Pericardium meridian; SI = Small Intestine meridian; Sp = Spleen meridian; St = Stomach meridian; TW = Triple Warmer meridian; UB = Urinary Bladder meridian.

Figure 3-2. Normal energy flow through meridians during the day and night.

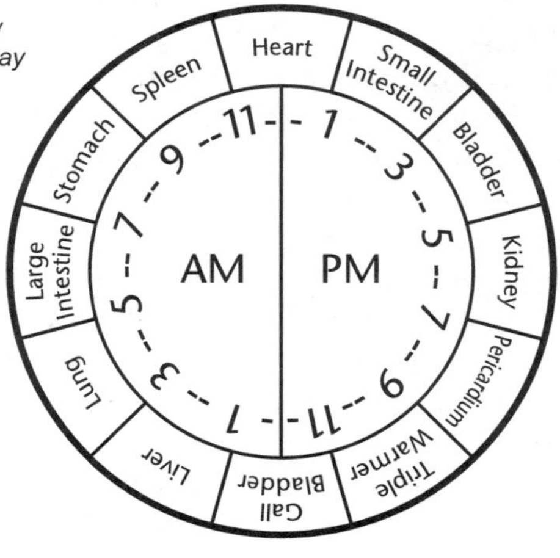

symptoms from other meridians. Some patients with blockage in one meridian can demonstrate just one symptom from the list, but it may be with great intensity. Some patients, even though they have energy disturbances in multiple meridians, may not show any symptoms. Such patients might have a better immune system than others. Variations with all these possibilities can make diagnosis difficult in some cases.

For further study of the acupuncture meridians, please see the Bibliography under Basic Science: Oriental Medicine. In particular, *Essentials of Chinese Acupuncture* offers excellent information on this topic.

Symptoms of Meridians

The Lung Meridian (Lu)
Energy disturbance in the lung meridian affecting *physical and physiological* levels can give rise to the following symptoms:

Skin disorders:
- Atopic dermatitis
- Cradle cap
- Dry skin
- Eczema
- Hives - generalized
- Hair loss
- Hair thinning
- Infantile eczema
- Itching of the body, scalp, nose
- Moles
- Poor growth of nails and hair
- Rashes
- Red cheeks and eyes
- Scaly and rough skin
- Skin tags
- Warts
- White spots on the body

Also:
- Bronchiectasis
- Bronchitis
- Burning in the eyes, & nostrils
- Cardiac asthma
- Chest congestion & cough
- Coughing up blood
- Discharge (thick and yellow in bacterial infections; thin or thick and white in viral infections)
- Dry mouth and throat
- Emaciated look
- Emphysema
- Fever with chills
- Flu-like symptoms (frequent)
- General body ache with burning sensation
- Glands swollen in the neck
- Hay fever

- Headache between eyes
- Inability to sleep after 3 a.m.
- Infection in the respiratory tract
- Lack of desire to talk
- Laryngitis and pharyngitis
- Low voice
- Morning fatigue
- Nasal congestion or runny nose
- Night sweats
- Nose bleed
- Pain between third and fourth thoracic vertebrae
- Pain in the chest and intercostal muscles in the eyes
- Pain in the first interphalangeal joint and thumb
- Pain in the upper arms and back
- Pain in the upper first and second cuspids (teeth)
- Perspiration (lack or excessive)
- Pleurisy
- Pneumonia
- Postnasal drip
- Restlessness between 3 to 5 a.m.
- Sinus headaches and infection
- Sneezing
- Stuffy nose
- Tenosynovitis
- Throat irritation
- Throat mucus
- Throat soreness
- Throat swelling
- Tonsilitis

Energy disturbance in the lung meridian affecting the *cellular* level can cause the following symptoms. When one fails to cry, or when one feels deep sorrow, sadness will settle in the lungs and eventually cause various lung disorders.

- Apologizing
- Comparing self with others
- Contempt
- Dejection
- Depression
- Despair
- False pride
- Grief or sadness
- Highly sensitive emotionally
- Hopelessness
- Intolerance
- Likes to humiliate others
- Loneliness
- Low self-esteem
- Meanness
- Melancholy
- Over-demanding
- Over-sympathetic
- Prejudice
- Seeking approval from others
- Self pity
- Weeping frequently

The Large Intestine Meridian (LI)

Energy disturbance in the large intestine meridian affecting *physical and physiological* levels can give rise to the following symptoms:

Skin disorders:
- Acne on the face, sides of the mouth and nose
- Dermatitis
- Eczema
- Hives
- Itching of the body
- Moles
- Skin rashes
- Skin tags
- Warts on the skin

Also:
- Abdominal pain
- Arthritis of the index finger
- Arthritis of the knee joint
- Arthritis of the lateral part of the elbow and hip
- Arthritis of the shoulder joint
- Arthritis of the wrist joint
- Asthma after 5 a.m.
- Bad breath
- Blisters in the lower gum
- Bursitis
- Dry mouth and thirst
- Fatigue
- Feeling better after a bowel movement

- Feeling tired after a bowel movement
- Flatulence
- Headaches
- Inflammation of lower gum
- Intestinal colic
- Loose stools or constipation
- Lower backache
- Mental fog
- Motor impairment of the fingers
- Muscle spasms and pain of lateral aspect of thigh, knee and below knee
- Pain and swelling of the index finger
- Pain in the heel
- Pain in the knee
- Pain in the shoulder, shoulder blade and back of the neck
- Poor clarity in thinking
- Sciatic pain
- Sinusitis
- Swollen cervical glands
- Tennis elbow
- Tenosynovitis
- Toothache

Energy disturbance in the large intestine meridian affecting the *cellular* level can cause the following symptoms:

- Guilt
- Confusion
- Brain fog
- Bad dreams
- Dwelling on past memory
- Crying spells
- Defensiveness

- Inability to recall dreams
- Nightmares
- Nostalgia
- Rolling restlessly in sleep
- Seeking sympathy
- Talking in the sleep
- Weeping

The Stomach Meridian (St)

Energy disturbance in the stomach meridian affecting *physical and physiological* levels can give rise to the following symptoms:

Skin disorders:
- Acne (painful) in the upper front of the body
- Acne on the face and neck
- Black/blue marks on the leg below the knee
- Blemishes
- Fever blisters
- Herpes
- Itching on the skin
- Rashes

Also:
- Abdominal Pains & distention
- Acid reflux disorders
- ADD & ADHD
- Anorexia
- Autism
- Bad breath
- Bipolar disorder
- Bulimia
- Chest muscle pain
- Coated tongue
- Cold sores in the mouth
- Coldness in the lower limbs
- Delirium
- Depression
- Dry nostrils
- Dyslexia

- Excessive hunger
- Facial paralysis
- Fibromyalgia
- Flushed face
- Frontal headache
- Hiatal hernia
- High fever
- Insomnia due to nervousness
- Learning disability
- Manic-depressive disorders
- Migraine headaches
- Nasal polyps
- Nausea
- Nosebleed
- Pain in the eye
- Pain in the mid-back
- Pain on the upper jaws
- Seizures
- Sensitivity to cold
- Sore throat
- Sores on the gums & tongue
- Sweating
- Swelling on the neck
- Temporomandibular joint (TMJ) problem
- Unable to relax the mind
- Upper gum diseases
- Vomiting

Energy disturbance in the stomach meridian affecting the *cellular* level can cause the following symptoms:

- Aggressive behaviors
- Attention deficit disorders
- Bitterness
- Butterfly sensation in the stomach
- Disgust

The Spleen Meridian (Sp)

Energy disturbance in the spleen meridian affecting *physical and physiological* levels can give rise to the following symptoms:

Skin disorders:
- Bleeding under the skin
- Bruises under the skin
- Cold sores on the lips
- Generalized edema
- Purpura
- Varicose veins

Also:
- Abnormal smell
- Abnormal taste
- Abnormal uterine bleeding
- Absence of menstruation
- Alzheimer's disease
- Autism
- Bitter taste in the mouth
- Bleeding from the mucous membrane
- Carpal tunnel syndrome
- Chronic gastroenteritis
- Coldness of the legs
- Cramps after the first day of menses
- Depression
- Diabetes
- Dizzy spells
- Dreams that cause fatigue
- Emaciated muscles
- Failing memory
- Fatigue in general
- Fatigue of the mind
- Fatigued limbs
- Feverishness
- Fibromyalgia
- Fluttering of the eyelids
- Hard lumps in the abdomen
- Hemophilia
- Hemorrhoids
- Hyperglycemia
- Hypertension
- Hypoglycemia
- Inability to make decisions
- Incontinence of urine or stool
- Indigestion
- Infertility
- Insomnia (usually unable to fall asleep)
- Intuitive and prophetic behaviors
- Irregular periods
- Lack of enthusiasm
- Lack of interest in anything
- Lethargy
- Light-headedness
- Loose stools
- Nausea
- Numbness on fingers and hands
- Obesity
- Pain and stiffness of the fingers
- Pain anywhere in the body
- Pain in the great toes
- Pallor
- Pedal edema
- Pencil-like thin stools with undigested food particles
- Poor memory
- Prolapse of the bladder
- Prolapse of the uterus
- Reduced appetite
- Schizophrenia
- Sensation of heaviness in the body and head
- Sleep during the day
- Slowing of the mind
- Sluggishness
- Stiffness of the tongue
- Sugar craving
- Swelling anywhere in the body
- Swellings or pain with swelling of the toes and feet
- Swollen eyelids
- Swollen lips
- Tingling or abnormal sensation in the tip of the fingers and palms
- Vomiting
- Watery eyes

Energy disturbance in the spleen meridian affecting the *cellular* level can cause the following symptoms:

- Anxiety
- Concern
- Dislikes crowds
- Easily hurt
- Gives more importance to self
- Hopelessness
- Irritable
- Keeps feelings inside
- Lack of confidence
- Likes loneliness
- Likes to be praised
- Likes to take revenge
- Lives through others
- Low self-esteem
- Needs constant encouragement
- Obsessive-Ccompulsive behavior
- Over sympathetic to others
- Restrained
- Sand-like feeling in the eyes
- Scanty menstrual flow
- Shy/timid
- Talks to self
- Unable to make decisions
- Worry

The Heart Meridian (Ht)

Energy disturbance in the heart meridian affecting the *physical and physiological* level can cause the following symptoms:

Skin disorders:
- Acne
- Boils
- Hives
- Itching on the forehead
- Painful pimple near the inner canthus of the eye
- Red spots on the body

Also:
- Angina-like pains
- Chest pains
- Discomfort when reclining
- Dizziness
- Dry throat
- Excessive perspiration
- Feverishness
- Headache
- Heart palpitation
- Heaviness in the chest
- Hot palms and soles
- Insomnia (unable to fall asleep when awakened in the middle of sleep
- Irritability
- Mental disorders
- Nervousness
- Pain along the left arm
- Pain along the scapula
- Pain and fullness in the chest
- Pain in the eye
- Poor circulation
- Shortness of breath
- Shoulder pains

Energy disturbance in the heart meridian affecting the *cellular* level can cause the following symptoms:

- Abusive nature
- Aggression
- Anger
- Bad manners
- Compassion and love
- Compulsive behaviors
- Dislikes making friends
- Does not trust anyone
- Easily upset
- Excessive laughing or crying
- Guilt
- Hostility
- Insecurity
- Joy
- Lack of emotions
- Lack of love and compassion
- Overexcitement
- Sadness
- Self-confidence
- Type A personality

The Small Intestine Meridian (SI)

Energy disturbance in the small intestine meridian affecting *physical and physiological* levels can give rise to the following symptoms:

Skin disorders:
- Acne on the upper back

Also:
- Abdominal pain
- Abdominal fullness
- Bad breath
- Constipation
- Bitter taste in the mouth
- Diarrhea
- Distention of lower abdomen
- Dry stool
- Frozen shoulder
- Knee pain
- Night sweats
- Pain in the neck
- Numbness of the back of the shoulder and arm
- Shoulder pain
- Numbness of the mouth and tongue
- Sore throat
- Pain along the side of the shoulder and arm
- Stiff neck
- Pain radiating around the waist

Energy disturbance in the small intestine meridian affecting the *cellular* level can cause the following symptoms:

- Absentmindedness
- Becoming too involved with details
- Day dreaming
- Easily annoyed
- Emotional instability
- Excessive joy or lack of joy
- Feeling of abandonment
- Feeling shy
- Insecurity
- Irritability
- Lacking confidence
- Over excitement
- Paranoia
- Poor concentration
- Sadness
- Sighing
- Sorrow
- Suppressing deep sorrow
- Tendency to be introverted and easily hurt

The Urinary Bladder Meridian (UB)

Energy disturbance in the Urinary Bladder meridian affecting *physical and physiological* levels can give rise to the following symptoms:

Skin disorders:
- Jock itch
- Psoriasis along the course of the meridian (especially along the vertebrae)
- Rashes

Also:
- Arthritis of little finger and toe
- Bloody urine
- Burning or painful urination
- Chills and fever
- Disease of the eye
- Frequent urination
- Headaches at the back of the neck
- Loss of bladder control
- Lower abdominal discomfort
- Lower back ache and stiffness
- Mental disorders
- Muscle wasting
- Nasal congestion
- Pain along the meridian
- Pain and/or spasms along back of the leg, foot, and lateral part of the sole and toes
- Pain in the ankle (lateral part)
- Pain in the inner canthus
- Retention of urine
- Sciatic neuralgia
- Spasm behind the knee
- Spasms of the calf muscles
- Stiff neck
- Weakness in the rectum and rectal muscle

Energy disturbance in the urinary bladder meridian affecting the *cellular* level can cause the following symptoms:

- Annoyed
- Disturbing and impure thoughts
- Fearful
- Fright
- Frustrated
- Highly irritable
- Impatient
- Inefficient
- Insecure
- Reluctant
- Restless
- Sadness
- Unhappy

The Kidney Meridian (Kid)

Energy disturbance in the kidney meridian affecting *physical and physiological* levels can give rise to the following symptoms:

Skin disorders:
- Acne
- Cradle cap
- Eczema
- Fungal infection
- Hair loss
- Itching

Also:
- Asthma (mild but nagging)
- Bags under the eyes
- Blurred vision
- Burning or painful urination
- Chronic diarrhea
- Cold feet
- Coldness in the back
- Crave salt
- Dark circles under the eyes
- Dryness of the mouth
- Ear pain
- Excessive salivation
- Excessive sleeping
- Excessive thirst
- Facial edema
- Fatigue
- Fever with chills
- Foot pain (on the sole)
- Frequent urination
- Impotence
- Irritability
- Leg pain (posterior aspect of leg or thigh)
- Light-headedness
- Lower back ache
- Motor impairment
- Muscular atrophy of the foot
- Nausea
- Poor appetite
- Poor concentration
- Poor memory
- Puffy eyes
- Ringing in the ears
- Sore throat
- Spasms of the ankle and feet
- Swelling in the legs
- Swollen ankles and vertigo

Energy disturbance in the kidney meridian affecting the
cellular level can cause the following symptoms:

- Caution
- Confused
- Fear
- Indecision

- Paranoia
- Seeks attention
- Terror
- Unable to express feelings

The Pericardium Meridian (Pc)

Energy disturbance in the pericardium meridian affecting
physical and physiological levels can give rise to the following
symptoms:

Skin disorders:
- Hives
- Red rashes on the chest

Also:
- Chest pain
- Contracture of the arm or elbow
- Excessive appetite
- Fainting spells
- Flushed face
- Frozen shoulder
- Fullness in the chest
- Heaviness in the chest
- Hot palms and soles
- Impaired speech

- Irritability
- Motor impairment of the tongue
- Nausea
- Nervousness
- Pain in the anterior part of the thigh
- Pain in the eyes
- Pain in the medial part of the knee
- Palpitation
- Restricting movements
- Sensation of hot or cold
- Slurred speech
- Spasms of the elbow and arm

Energy disturbance in the pericardium meridian affecting the
cellular level can cause the following symptoms:

- Extreme joy
- Fear of heights
- Heaviness in the chest due to emotional overload
- Heaviness in the head
- Hurt
- Imbalance in sexual energy
- In some cases no desire for sex
- Jealousy

- Light sleep with dreams
- Manic disorders
- Over- excitement
- Regret
- Sexual coldness
- Sexual tension
- Shock
- Stubbornness
- Various phobias

The Triple Warmer Meridian (TW)

Energy disturbance in the triple warmer meridian affecting *physical and physiological* levels can give rise to the following symptoms:

Skin disorders:
- Acne
- Hives on the chest and abdomen
- Pimples on the chest

Also:
- Abdominal pain
- Always feels hungry even after eating a full meal
- Constipation
- Deafness
- Distention
- Dysuria
- Edema
- Enuresis
- Excessive hunger
- Excessive thirst
- Fever in the late evening
- Frequent urination
- Hardness and fullness in the lower abdomen
- Indigestion
- Pain behind the ear
- Pain in the cheek and jaw
- Pain in the medial part of the knee
- Pain in the shoulder and upper arm
- Redness in the eye
- Shoulder pain
- Swelling and pain in the throat
- Vertigo

Energy disturbance in the triple warmer meridian affecting the *cellular* level can cause the following symptoms:

- Depression
- Deprivation
- Despair
- Emptiness
- Excessive emotion
- Grief
- Hopelessness
- Phobias

The Gall Bladder Meridian (GB)

Energy disturbance in the gall bladder meridian affecting *physical and physiological* levels can give rise to the following symptoms:

Skin disorders:
- Black heads on the face
- Dry skin
- Eczema
- Hair loss
- Itching all over the body
- Shingles

Also:
- Abdominal bloating
- Alternating fever and chills
- Ashen complexion
- Bitter taste in the mouth
- Burping after meals
- Chills
- Deafness
- Dizziness
- Fever
- Headaches on the sides of the head
- Heartburn after fatty foods
- Heavy sensation in the right upper part of the abdomen
- Hyperacidity
- Moving arthritis
- Nausea with fried foods
- Pain and cramps along the front right or left side of the abdomen
- Pain in the eye
- Pain in the hip
- Pain in the jaw
- Poor digestion of fats
- Sciatic neuralgia
- Sighing
- Stroke-like condition
- Swelling under the jaw
- Tremors
- Twitching
- Vision disturbances
- Vomiting
- Yellowish complexion

Energy disturbance in the gall bladder meridian affecting the *cellular* level can cause the following symptoms:

- Aggression
- Complaining all the time
- Fearful
- Judgmental
- Rage
- Unhappiness

The Liver Meridian (Liv)

Energy disturbance in the liver meridian affecting *physical and physiological* levels can give rise to the following symptoms:

Skin disorders:
- Brown spots on the skin
- Dry skin
- Dry, parched, or cracking lips
- Itching all over the body

Also:
- Abdominal pain
- Blurred vision
- Bright colored bleeding during menses
- Dark urine
- Dizziness
- Enuresis
- Feeling of obstruction in the throat
- Fever
- Hard lumps in the upper abdomen
- Headache at the top of the head
- Hemiplegia
- Hernia
- Irregular menses
- Jaundice
- Loose stools
- Pain in the breasts
- Pain in the intercostal region
- Pain in the lower abdomen
- Paraplegia
- Premenstrual syndrom (PMS)
- Reproductive organ disturbances
- Retention of urine
- Seizures
- Spasms in the extremities
- Stroke-like condition
- Tinnitus
- Vertigo
- Vomiting

Energy disturbance in the liver meridian affecting the *cellular* level can cause the following symptoms:

- Aggression
- Anger
- Assertion
- Irritability
- Rage
- Shouting
- Talking loud
- Type A personality

The Governing Vessel Meridian (GV)

The governing vessel meridian supplies the brain and spinal region, running along with the spine from the back of the body, so it connects with all 31 spinal nerve roots, connects with all 12 meridians, and also connects with the conception vessel meridian at the lip.

Energy disturbance in the governing vessel meridian affecting *physical, physiological, and psychological* levels can give rise to the following symptoms:

- Certain mental disorders
- Colic
- Constipation
- Fevers
- Functional infertility
- Heavy sensation in the head
- Hemorrhoids
- Involuntary urination
- Shaking
- Stiffness and pain along the spinal column
- Vertigo
- Various mixed symptoms of other meridians

The Conception Vessel Meridian (CV)

The conception vessel meridian travels through the midline of front of the body from the pubis to the lip, then encircles the mouth, and goes to the eyes. It connects with all 12 meridians on the front of the body; with its function closely related with pregnancy, it has intimate links with the kidneys and uterus.

Energy disturbance in the conception vessel meridian affecting *physical, physiological, and psychological* levels can give rise to the following symptoms:

- Colic
- Impotency
- Irregular menstruation
- Leukorrhea
- Low libido
- Male and female infertility
- Urogenital system disorders
- Various mixed symptoms of other meridians, especially liver and kidney

NAET® DIAGNOSTIC APPROACH

The NAET® approach is a unique blend of conventional Western (allopathic) medical approaches, Oriental medical approaches, and Applied Kinesiologic methods. With this approach, it is extremely important for the patient to cooperate with the NAET® Specialist in order to obtain the best results. This section is designed to help promote an understanding between NAET® Specialists and their patients because, in order to obtain the most satisfactory results, both parties must work together as a team.

Medical History

The first step in diagnosing a skin problem is to take a thorough patient history, including chief complaint, present history, past medical history, family history, social history, history of activities, hobbies, pets, travel, nutrition, and drug ingestion (including over-the-counter medicines). Patients are given a symptom survey form to record the level and type of discomfort. It is helpful to obtain a thorough record of any past sensitivity reactions in the patient's family, tracing back two or three generations if possible. The patient will be asked whether either parent suffers from eczema or hay fever, ever suffered from hives, reacted to a serum injection (such as tetanus anti-toxin, DPT), or experienced any type of skin trouble. Additionally, the NAET® Specialist will ask whether the patient's parents were unable to eat certain foods or professed to "hate" certain foods because of how the particular food made them feel; complained of itching, hives, sinusitis, runny nose, frequent colds or flu; had dyspepsia, indigestion, mental illness, heart disorders, any other skin disorders, foot ulcers, yeast infections, frequent choking sensation, throat closing-like sensation or any other conditions where an allergy may have been a contributing factor, whether or not recognized as such at the time.

The same questions are asked about the patient's other relatives: grandparents, aunts, uncles, brothers, sisters, and cousins. An allergic tendency is not always inherited directly from the parents. It may skip generations, and often manifest in nieces or nephews rather than in direct descendants.

The careful NAET® Specialist will also determine whether such diseases as tuberculosis, cancer, diabetes, rheumatic or glandular disorders exist or have ever occurred in the patient's family history. All of these facts help give the NAET® Specialist a more complete picture of the patient's hereditary factors. Allergic tendency is inherited, though it may be manifested differently in different people. Unlike the tendency, an actual allergic condition such as eczema is not always inherited. Parents may have had diabetes or rheumatism, but the child can manifest that allergic inheritance as general body itching, skin rashes, acne, eczema, or other skin related symptom.

When the family history is complete, the NAET® Specialist will need to look into the patient's recent history of dermatological reactions. Some typical preliminary questions include: "When did your first episode occur? Did your eczema first occur when you were an infant or a child, or did you first notice the symptoms of eczema after you were fully grown? Did it occur after going through a certain procedure? For example, did it occur for the first time after a course of antibiotics for a throat infection?"

One of my patients reported that her eczema began after completing a course of antibiotics that she had taken for a severe throat infection (strep-throat). She was found to be allergic to Streptococcus pyogenus *bacteria as well as to the antibiotics.*

Once a careful history is taken, the NAET® Specialist often discovers that the patient's first symptoms occurred in early childhood. He or she may have suffered from skin rashes, diaper rash, or infantile eczema, but never associated it with allergic contact dermatitis, which may not have appeared until later when he/she used the special herbal shampoo.

Next, the NAET® Specialist will want to know the circumstances surrounding and immediately preceding the first symptoms. Typical questions will include: "Did you change your diet or go on a special diet? Did you eat something that you hadn't eaten perhaps for two or three months? Do you eat one type of food repeatedly, every day? Did the symptoms follow a childhood illness (whooping cough, measles, chicken pox, diphtheria) or any immunization for such an illness? Did they follow some other illness, such as influenza, pneumonia, viral infection, or a major operation? Did the symptoms first appear at adolescence or after you had a baby? Were they first noticed after you acquired a cat, a dog, or even a bird? Did they appear after an automobile accident or any major physical or mental trauma? Did they appear after a lengthly exposure to the sun, a day at the beach, or 18 holes of golf? Did they appear after receiving a gift for your birthday? Or after starting to use a new pair of shoes, slippers, socks, pants, shirt, after-shave, wrist watch, leather belt, leather shoes, chair, furniture, certain shampoo, cosmetics, after using certain chemicals in the carpet cleaning process, or after installing a new carpet? Did your symptoms begin after a new arrival in the house (a baby, a guest, a pet, etc.)?"

Any one of these factors can be responsible for triggering a severe allergic manifestation on the skin, or precipitate the first noticeable symptoms of an allergic condition. Therefore, it is very important to obtain full and accurate answers when taking a patient's medical history.

Other important questions also should relate to the frequency and occurrence of the sensitivity-reaction episodes. Although foods may be a factor, if the symptoms occur only at specific times of the year, the trouble is most likely due to pollens. Often a patient is sensitive to certain foods but has a natural tolerance that prevents sickness until the pollen sensitivity adds sufficient allergens to throw the body into an imbalance. If itching and scratching occur only on specific days of the week, they are probably due to something contacted or eaten on that particular day.

The causes of allergic attacks in different patients can, at first, appear to be random, as seen in the following case. *Regular weekly attacks of hives and skin rashes were the effects in one patient after he walked in the park twice a week for 30 minutes. The grass or something on the grass (pesticides perhaps) caused this allergic reaction. Another patient reacted similarly to the walk in the park. He always sat on the bench at the end of his walk and always came home with hives in exposed skin surface. Other cases demonstrate this point as well. A man always had severe abdominal distention and skin rashes whenever he ate anything that contained tomato. He was allergic to tomatoes. Still another patient had an allergic attack of hives and runny nose on Saturdays. I traced the allergy to the chemical compounds in a lotion she used to set her hair on Friday afternoons.*

The time of day when the episodes occur is also of importance in determining the cause of an allergic manifestation. If it always occurs at night, it is quite likely that there is something in the bedroom that is aggravating the condition. It may be that the patient is sensitive to feathers in the pillow or comforter, wood cabinets, marble floors, carpets, side tables, end tables, bed sheets, pillows, pillow cases, detergents used in washing clothes, indoor plants, or shrubs, trees or grasses outside the patient's window.

Many patients react violently to house dust, different types of furniture, polish, houseplants, tap water, and purified water, causing eczema reactions of varying intensities. Most city water suppliers change the water chemicals once or twice a year. This is done with good intentions: people with chemical allergies may become more sick if they ingest the same chemicals over and over for months or years. Changing chemicals like chlorine to chloramine and back to chlorine every six months gives an opportunity for the chemically sensitive person not to be continuously exposed to the same chemical throughout the year.

I knew certain patients reacted to city water throughout the year and suffered from weeping eczema all over the body. Until they were treated with NAET® for chlorine and chloramine, they continued to suffer from their incurable skin disorders that did not respond to any medication. Contrary to traditional Western thinking, developing immunity can be the exception rather than the rule.

Occasionally, switching foods, chemicals or other substances gives a change of allergens to an allergic patient and a chance for him/her to recover from reactions. In this way, some allergic reactions can be avoided.

The NAET® Specialist should ask the patient to make a daily log of all the foods he/she is eating and all other daily activities. The ingredients in the food should be checked for possible allergens. Certain common allergens like food chemicals, corn products, MSG (monosodium glutamate or Accent®), citric acid, etc., are used in many food preparations.

A number of food chemicals are used in the food industry. People who tend to have dermatological problems often experience itching and dermatitis when they consume ready-made and packaged foods with these food chemicals and additives. A few such food chemicals are: acetic acid, agar, albumin, aldicarb, alginates, propylene glycol, aluminum salts, sodium aluminum phosphate, benzoates, calcium propionate, calcium silicate, carbamates, carbon monoxide, EDTA, ethylene gas, food bleach, formic acid, malic acid, mannan, mannitol, salicylic acid, succinic acid, talc, tartaric acid, and various water pollutants.

Allergy to corn is one of today's most common allergies, especially in chemically sensitive patients. Unfortunately, cornstarch is found in almost every processed food, some toiletries, and even in drugs. Chinese food, baking soda, baking powder and toothpaste contain large amounts of cornstarch. It is the binding product in almost all vitamins and pills, including Aspirin® and Tylenol®. Corn syrup is the natural sweetener in many of the products we ingest, including soft drinks. Corn silk is found in cosmetics, and corn oil is used as a vegetable oil. Cotton crotches of female underpants are treated with baking soda and baking powder for better hygiene. But an allergy to corn from baking soda is found to be one of the common sources of never-ending yeast-like infections in chemically sensitive women. Many women became free of yeast-like infections after treating with NAET® for cornstarch.

People react severely to various gums used in many preparations, including acacia gum, xanthine gum, and karaya gum. Numerous gums are used in a variety of foods, such as candy bars, yogurt, cream cheese, soft drinks, soy sauce, barbecue sauce, fast food products, and macaroni and cheese.

Exposure to any of these items can produce debilitating skin symptoms. Very often the diagnosis is based on symptoms alone, and the original cause of sensitivity is overlooked.

Physical Examination

The history should be followed by a thorough clinical examination, including observation of the mental status, face, skin, eyes, color, posture, movements, gait, tongue, scars, wounds, marks, and body secretions. The area(s) of the complaints, as well as distribution and manifestation of the condition, should be evaluated thoroughly. Evaluation of blood pressure, pulse, skin temperature, and palpable pains in the course of meridians should be done. The combination of thorough medical history and physical examination should help form a working clinical diagnosis.

Laboratory Tests

Laboratory investigations of allergic diseases should not be considered without a detailed clinical history and a working clinical diagnosis. Properly selected, laboratory confirmation of an allergy (see Western Medicine Diagnostic Approach above) is specific, safe for the patient, and provides a quantitative level for specific IgE which may be important for follow-up purposes. If the NAET® Specialist is not able to perform these tests, the patient should be referred to an appropriate specialist or facility that can perform the tests and send results to the NAET® Specialist.

Instrument Tests

Skin Resistance Test (SRT)

A Skin Resistance Test (SRT) — also called the ElectroDermal Test (EDT) — may be used to detect the presence or absence of a suspected allergen. This computerized testing device provides meter readings; differences in the meter reading are observed, and the greater differences in readings indicate the stronger allergies.

Dynamometer Testing

A hand-held dynamometer is used to measure finger strength (0-100 scale) in the presence and absence of a suspected allergen. The dynamometer is held with thumb and index finger and squeezed to make the reading needle swing between 0-100 scale.

An initial base-line reading is observed first, then the allergen is held and another reading taken. The finger strength is compared in the presence of the allergen. If the second reading is more than the initial reading, there is no allergy. If the second reading is less than the initial reading, then there is an allergy.

Pulse Test

The Pulse test is another simple way to determine food allergy. This method was developed by Arthur Coca, M.D. in the 1950s. Research has shown that if a person is allergic to something and eats it, the pulse rate increases. The subject's baseline pulse is established by counting the radial pulse (on the thumb side of the wrist) for a full minute. Then a small portion of the suspected allergen is put in the subject's mouth, preferably under the tongue. The subject should taste the substance for two minutes, without swallowing any portion of it. The taste will send the signal to the brain, which will send a signal through the sympathetic nervous system to the rest of the body. *(Important note: If the subject is known or suspected to be severely allergic to the item, the item should not be put in the mouth. Instead, it should just be held in the hand by touching with the finger pads, which are as sensitive as putting it in the mouth.)* The pulse is then taken again with the allergen still in the mouth (or in the hand, as noted above). An increase or decrease in pulse rate of 10% or more is considered an allergic reaction. A greater difference in the pulse rate indicates a greater the degree of allergy. This is a useful test for food allergies.

Oriental Medicine and Applied Kinesiology

In Oriental medicine theory, the flow and balance of vital energy or life force is necessary to maintain health. Energy medicine maintains that the pool of electromagnetic energy around an object or a person allows for an energy exchange: the human field absorbs the energy from the nearby object, and processes it through the network of nerve energy pathways. If the foreign energy field shares suitable charges with the human energy field, the human field absorbs the foreign energy for its advantage and becomes stronger. If the foreign energy field carries unsuitable charges, the human energy field causes repulsion of the foreign energy field, and the substance itself is considered an allergen to the particular individual. People frequently go near allergens and interact with their energies without recognizing this repulsive action, whether from foods, drinks, chemicals, environmental substances, animals or other humans. This causes energy disturbances in the meridians; thereby causing imbalances in the body. The imbalances cause illnesses, which create disorganization in body functions most often leading to hives, itching, edema, eczema, acne, candidiasis, other skin problems, or other health problems. The disorganization of the body and its functions involve the vital organs, their associated muscle groups, and nerve roots, which can give rise to brain disorders. To prevent the allergen from causing further disarray after producing the initial blockage, the brain sends messages to every cell of the body to reject the presence of the allergen. This rejection will appear as repulsion, and the repulsion will produce different symptoms related to the affected organs.

Neuromuscular sensitivity testing (NST) is the body's communication pathway to the brain, and is based on the principles of *I Ching*, a 6,000-year-old Chinese diagnostic modality. It is also closely related to MRT (muscle response testing), a standard test used in Applied Kinesiology, which originated with Dr. George Goodheart and his associates and has been practiced in the United States since 1964. (For more information, see the Bibliography sections on Applied Kinesiology, and Basic Science: Oriental Medicine.)

NAET® NEUROMUSCULAR SENSITIVITY TESTING (NST)

Neuromuscular sensitivity testing (NST) is one of the tools used by NAET® Specialists to test imbalances and allergies in the body, as well as to detect various allergens that cause imbalances in the body. This method compares the strength of a predetermined muscle (PDM) in the presence and absence of a suspected allergen. If the particular muscle (test muscle) weakens in the presence of an item, it signifies that the item is an allergen. If the muscle remains strong, the substance is not an allergen. Neuromuscular sensitivity testing can be performed in the following ways:

1. Standard NST can be done in laying down, standing, or sitting positions (Figures 3-3 through 3-8).
2. The "Oval Ring" test can be used on a very strong person with a strong arm (Figures 3-9 through 3-10).
3. Surrogate testing can be used to test an infant, disabled or very weak person, or an extremely strong person (Figures 3-11 through 3-13).

Standard NST Procedure

Two people are required to perform standard neuromuscular sensitivity testing: the tester, and the subject.

Step 1: Figure 3-3 shows the subject laying on a firm surface with the left arm raised 45-90 degrees to the body with the palm facing outward and the thumb pointing toward the big toe.

Step 2: The tester stands on the subject's (right) side. The subject's right arm is kept to his/her side with the palm either kept open to the air, or in a loose fist. The fingers should not touch any material, fabric, or any part of the table on which the arm is resting because this can confuse the test results. The tester's left palm is contacting the subject's left wrist.

Step 3: It is essential to test a strong predetermined muscle (PDM) to get accurate results. The tester using the left arm tries to push the raised arm toward the subject's left big toe. The subject resists the push. The arm, or predetermined indicator muscle, remains strong if the subject is well balanced at the time of testing. If the muscle or raised arm is weak and gives way under pressure without the presence of an allergen, either the subject is not balanced, or the tester is performing the test improperly; for example, the tester might be trying to overpower the subject. The subject does not need to gather up strength from other muscles in the body to resist the tester. Only five to ten pounds of pressure need to be applied for three to five seconds. If the muscle shows weakness, the tester will be able to judge the difference with only that small amount of pressure.

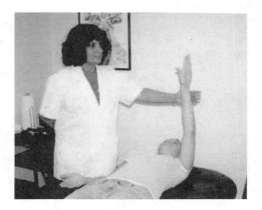

Figure 3-3. Initial NST without allergen.

Step 4: This step is used if the patient is found to be out of balance as indicated by the PDM presenting weak without the presence of an allergen. Figure 3-4 shows the tester using the balancing points by placing the fingertips of right hand at Point 1, and the fingertips of the left hand at Point 2. The tester massages these two points gently clockwise with the fingertips for 30-60 seconds, and then repeats steps 2 and 3 (above). If the PDM tests weak, the tester repeats Step 4 until the PDM becomes strong; in a very sick individual it may be necessary to repeat this procedure for three or four times before the

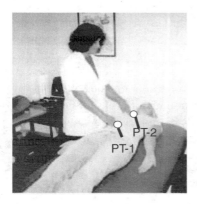

Figure 3-4. Initial balancing.

Point 1. *This point, called "Sea of Energy", is located two finger-breadths below the navel, on the midline. According to Oriental medical theory, this is where the energy of the body is stored in abundance. When the body senses any danger around its energy field or when the body experiences energy disturbances, the energy supply is cut short and stored here. If that energy reservoir point is massaged in a clockwise direction, the energy will come out of this storage and travel to Point 2.*

Point 2. *This point, called "Dominating Energy", is located in the center of the chest on the midline of the body, level with the fourth intercostal space. This is the energy dispenser department. According to Oriental medical theory, when the energy rises from the Sea of Energy (Point 1), it goes straight to the Dominating Energy point (Point 2). This is the point that controls and regulates the energy circulation or Chi flow in the body. From this point, the energy is distributed to different meridians, organs, tissues, and cells as needed to help remove the energy disturbances in those affected areas.*

PDM becomes strong. When the PDM tests strong, the tester continues with step 5.

Step 5: If the PDM remains strong when tested — a sign that the subject is balanced — then the tester should put the suspected allergen into the palm of the subject's resting hand (Figure 3-5). When the subject's fingertips touch the allergen, the sensory receptors sense the allergen's charges and relay the message to the brain. If it is an incompatible charge, the strong PDM will go weak (Figure 3-6). If the charges are compatible to the body, the PDM will remain strong (Figure 3-5). This way, the tester can check any number of items to determine the compatible and incompatible charges.

The subject can also be tested in a standing position (Figure 3-7) or sitting position (Figure 3-8). However, the laying-down

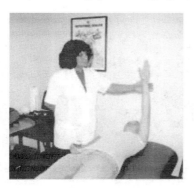

Figure 3-5. Standard NST with allergen.

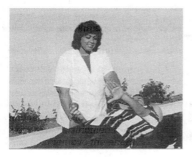

Figure 3-6. Standard NST weak with allergen.

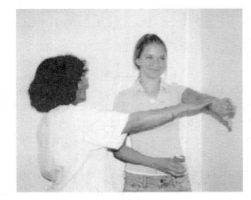

Figure 3-7. Standard NST with allergen – standing position.

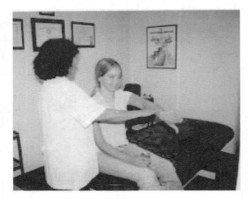

Figure 3-8. Standard NST with allergen – sitting position.

position is the most convenient for both tester and subject; it also achieves more accurate results.

"Oval Ring" NST Procedure

The "Oval Ring" test (also called "O Ring" test can be used to test a subject who has a strong arm, that is, if the subject is physically very strong and the tester is physically weak. (Note: This can also be used in self-testing after receiving NAET® Basic allergen treatments and practicing this method with guidance from a NAET® Specialist. For more information on self-testing, please see the end of this chapter.)

Step 1: Without any contact with an allergen, the subject makes an "O" shape by opposing the little finger and thumb on the same hand (finger pad to finger pad). Then, with the index finger of the other hand he/she tries to separate the "O Ring" against pressure (Figure 3-9). If the ring separates easily, the subject needs to be balanced, as described above.

Step 2: If the "O Ring" remains inseparable and strong, the subject holds an allergen in the other hand, by the fingertips, and performs step 1 again. If the "O Ring" separates easily, the substance in the hand is an allergen for that person. If the "O Ring" remains strong, the substance is not an allergen.

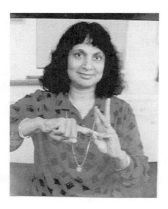

Figure 3-9. "O Ring" NST.

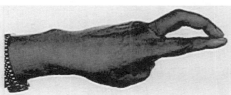

Figure 3-10. Finger-on-finger variation of "O Ring" NST.

A variation of this test is the finger-on-finger position (Figure 3-10). The strength of the muscles between these two fingers on the same hand is used to test and compare the strength without and with holding an allergen. The middle finger is pushed down, using the index finger of the same hand, or vice versa, in the absence and presence of the allergen in the other hand.

Surrogate NST Procedure

This method can be very useful to test and determine the allergies of an infant, a child, a hyperactive child, an autistic child, a disabled or very weak person, an unconscious person, or an extremely strong person.

Three people are required to perform surrogate NST: the tester, the subject, and the surrogate.

Step 1: Figures 3-11 and 3-12 show the *surrogate* laying on a firm surface with the left arm raised 45-90 degrees to the body with the palm facing outward and the thumb pointing toward the big toe.

Step 2: The tester stands on the right side of the surrogate, and the subject sits on the left side. The surrogate holds the allergen, while the subject touches the surrogate. As the tester performs NST using the surrogate's muscle (using the same procedure as in standard NST steps 2 and 3 above), it is very important that skin-to-skin contact is maintained between the surrogate and the subject during the procedure; if not, then the surrogate will receive the results of testing and treatment.

(Note: NAET® treatments can also be administered very effectively through the surrogate or extended surrogate without causing any interference in that surrogate's energy.)

Extended surrogate testing may be used when the subject is uncooperative, i.e., hyperactive, autistic, or frightened; this meth-

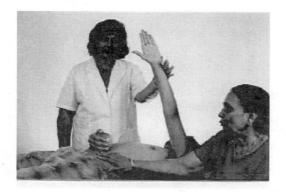

Figure 3-11. Surrogate NST.

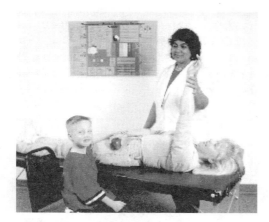

Figure 3-12. Surrogate NST – testing a toddler.

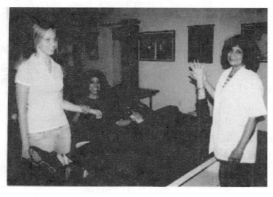

Figure 3-13. Extended surrogate NST.

od requires four people (Figure 3-13). As the tester performs NST using the surrogate's muscle, again, it is very important that skin-to-skin contact is maintained among the subject, the surrogate, and the extended surrogate. Testing or treatment does not affect the surrogates as long as the subject maintains uninterrupted skin-to-skin contact with the adjacent surrogate.

Testing Person-to-Person Allergies

NST can be used to test any substance for allergies, and even human beings can be tested for each other in this manner. A person who is allergic to another person (e.g., father, mother, son, daughter, grandfather, grandmother, spouse, caretaker, baby sitter) could experience symptoms similar to those experienced with foods, chemicals, or materials. If one person is allergic to another, the allergy can affect either person in various ways. If the father and/or mother is allergic to the child, or child allergic to a parent or parents, the child can become sick or remain sick indefinitely. If the husband is allergic to the wife or the wife is allergic to the husband, they might fight all the time and/or their health can be affected. The same things can happen among other family members. It is important to test family members and other immediate people in the patient's life for possible allergy, and if found, they should be receive NAET® treatment for each other (see Chapter 4).

Person-to-Person Allergy Testing Procedure
The subject lies down and touches the other person he or she wants tested (Figures 3-12 and 3-13). The tester pushes the arm of the subject, as with standard NST steps 2 and 3 above. If the subject is allergic to the other person, the indicator muscle goes weak. If the subject is not allergic, the indicator muscle remains strong. This is done through a surrogate in autistic children. Sometimes, one needs to test an autistic or hyperactive child through an ex-

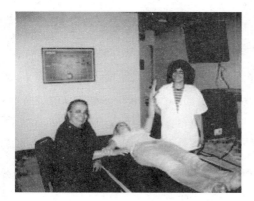

Figure 3-14. Person-to-Person NST for subject's allergy to another person.

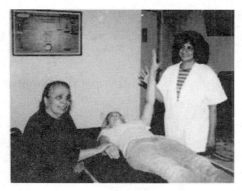

Figure 3-15. Person-to-Person NST for another person's allergy to subject.

tended surrogate because the child may be violent or too strong for one surrogate to handle.

NAET® QUESTION RESPONSE TESTING (QRT)

The brain and nervous system work around the clock to take care of the body's needs: they are watching and protecting from any physical, physiological, and/or emotional harm. The electromagnetically sensitive nervous system is very efficient in communicating with each nerve cell in the body in complete coordination, and also has the ability to connect and communicate with the electromagnetic forces of other living or nonliving beings of the universe from any distance. So, the brain can be trusted to find the best answers to questions about a person's health. Believe it or not, the brain never lies.

In other words, a person can ask his/her brain any question, and it will give the correct answer related to that person's health. Each cell in the brain and the nervous system is built uniquely with specialized cell materials that have the ability to measure and assess the energy differences of various factors in a person's internal and external environments, such as disturbed body functions, substances from our environment causing energy blockages, emotional disturbances, vibrations, temperature change that disturbs our energy flow or circulation in the body, and so on. A person (the subject) can be tested through a surrogate by asking these specific questions as long as the surrogate and the subject maintain skin-to-skin contact. This sharing ability of each nerve cell creates an excellent communication network system. This specialized communication is made possible for the nerve cell by its unique ability to transfer its electromagnetic energy in and out of the cell: within the body, out of the body, and to a distance of infinity.

Subconscious and conscious minds are part of the brain. The conscious mind thinks, feels, becomes tired or sleepy, etc., whereas the subconscious mind never thinks, becomes tired, or sleeps. A person's subconscious mind gathers information about everything regarding his/her health, and stores the information in the memory bank. So, a person's subconscious mind knows everything that has happened to that person from day one of his/her life. Subconscious mind records every bit of knowledge that is collected during a person's life, and stores it safely to recall in the future if it ever becomes necessary. The NAET® QRT method pulls information back out from this storage to help improve health.

NAET® QRT Procedure

It is best for a subject to be tested through a surrogate until self-testing procedures are learned and sufficiently practiced; then, this method can also be used for self-testing.

Step 1: Make a list of questions that need to be asked about the subject's health. Questions should be asked about the possible cause for the present health problem, the best treatment approach, etc. It is important to note that the subconscious brain accessed in this technique cannot talk in words or sentences; instead, ways must be created to extract answers from the brain for communication. (See "Techniques of Asking Questions".)

Step 2: Follow Steps 1 and 2 in the Surrogate NST Procedure. While subject and surrogate maintain skin-to-skin contact, the tester silently (in the mind) asks questions about the subject's health while testing the surrogate's PDM for its weakening or strengthening effect. (Rather than using a sample food or allergenic substance to check for weakening or strengthening effect, in QRT, the question becomes the "sample".) If the PDM is weak, the answer is interpreted as "yes." If the PDM tests strong, the answer is a "no."

The Techniques of Asking Questions

It may help to look at some examples of questions to use while performing QRT, such as with an 8-year-old child, Mark, who has been suffering from severe body eczema for the past two months. Mark is itching severely, bleeding almost all over his body, and he is fatigued, angry, and highly irritable. Using the NAET®-QRT procedure, the questions and responses might go something like this:

Question: Is your present health problem triggered by an allergy?

At the end of the question, the tester performs NST on the surrogate's PDM. If the PDM goes weak, Mark's subconscious mind is conveying the answer through the surrogate's muscle, "Yes, my present health problem is triggered by an allergy." If the PDM remains strong, then the child's subconscious mind is saying, "No, my present health problem is not triggered by an allergy."

If the PDM went weak in this case, the questions could continue as follows.

Question: If your problem is triggered by an allergy, is that allergen a solid food?
Answer: *Strong PDM indicates, "No, my problem is not triggered by a solid food."*

Question: "Is your problem triggered by a liquid that you drink?"
Answer: *Weak NST indicates a "Yes, It is a liquid."*

Question: "If it is caused by drinking a liquid, do you drink this liquid daily?"
Answer: *Weak NST indicates, "Yes, I drink this liquid daily."*

Question: "If you drink this liquid daily, is it milk?"
Answer: *Strong NST indicates, "No, it is not milk."*

Question: "If you drink this liquid daily, is it fruit juice?"
Answer: *Strong NST indicates, "No, it is not fruit juice."*

Question: "If you drink this liquid daily, is it soup?"
Answer: *Strong NST indicates, "No, it is not soup."*

Question: "If you drink this liquid daily, is it any liquid
             medication?"
Answer: *Strong NST indicates, "No, it is not liquid medication."*

Question: "If you drink this liquid daily, is it bottled water?"
Answer: *Strong NST indicates, "No, it is not bottled water."*

Question: "If you drink this liquid daily, is it tap water?"
Answer: *Weak NST indicates, "Yes, it is the tap water."*

Question: "Is the bathing in tap water causing your eczema?"
Answer: *Weak NST indicates, "Yes, it is causing my eczema."*

Question: "Is the drinking or bathing in tap water causing
             your itching?"
Answer: *Weak NST indicates, "Yes, it is causing my itching."*

Question: "Is the drinking of tap water causing your fatigue?"
Answer: *Weak NST indicates, "Yes, it is causing my fatigue."*

Question: "Are you allergic to the water from your city?"
Answer: *"No, I am not allergic to my city water."*

Question: "Is there something different in your tap water?"
Answer: *"Yes, there is something in my tap water."*

Question: "Are you allergic to the water filter salts we added two months ago?"

Answer: *"Yes, I am allergic to the water-filter salts we added two months ago."*

The questioning in this fashion suddenly brings to mind the water-filter salts that the family added to the water two months ago, just about that time Mark began itching, scratching, and developing this severe eczema that was nonresistant to all prescription medications, ointments, emollients and creams used on him for the past two months. If the child's conscious mind knew these answers then he would not have used the tap water for anything. His subconscious mind was the one giving you the answer.

In this example, the patient should take a sample of the tap water with filter-salts to the NAET® Specialist to treat Mark with NAET® for the tap water with the salt. Sometimes it may take more than one treatment just to desensitize for this one item. When the passes the treatment for the water, his symptoms will go away.

This QRT method should become part of every patient's routine to screen each food, drink, vitamin, medication, fabric, chemical, and of every other item from the surroundings the patient is exposed to the item(s). If all tested items are found to be allergens, then more items should be tested until a few nonallergic products can be found. These nonallergic products should be used exclusively until the allergic items are properly desensitized with NAET®.

NAET® SELF-TESTING

After receiving NAET® Basic allergen treatments from a trained NAET® practitioner (see Chapter 4), a patient can begin to test and screen daily encountered allergens before using them. Two methods used for self-testing are the "Oval Ring Test" or "O Ring Test" described in detail earlier in this chapter, and the Hold-Sit-Test method.

"O Ring" NST Method

NST is one of the most reliable methods of allergy tests, and it is fairly easy to learn and practice in every day life. The tester will develop confidence after enough practice. It can also reduce the need for expensive laboratory work. It is very important for people who are chemically sensitive to learn this simple testing technique to screen allergies before exposure, in order to prevent unexpected allergic reactions. Then the offending substances can easily be avoided, or if unavoidable, treated with NAET®. Because hundreds of new allergens enter the world daily (chemical manufacturers do not understand the predicament of allergic people), for an allergic person to live in this world looking and feeling normal, it is necessary to learn self-testing. It is not practical for anyone to treat thousands of allergens from their surroundings, or to go to a NAET® Specialist every day for the rest of one's life. Learning to detect the allergies on one's own, after treating for NAET® Basic allergens, makes it easier to avoid most other allergens by testing prior to exposures.

Much practice is needed to test and sense the differences properly. People should not become discouraged if they cannot do this properly or effectively the first few times; lots of practice will improve results.

A Tip to Master Self-Testing With "O Ring" NST

The following procedure can help a patient learn to sense the different between what is and what is not an allergen. Practicing this procedure will help the patient improve results when screening for daily-encountered allergens.

Step 1: The patient gathers two items, one that is a known allergen, and one that is not. For example, gather an apple (allergen) and a banana (non-allergen).

Step 2: The patient holds the apple (allergen) in the right hand, and does the "O Ring Test" as shown in Figure 3-9. The ring easily breaks. (If it does not break after the first few times, the subject should make it happen intentionally.)

Step 3: Then, the patient holds the banana (non-allergen), and performs the same test. This time the ring does not break.

Step 4: The patient puts the banana down, and rubs his/her hands together quickly for 30 seconds.

The patient should practice Steps 2-4 until he/she can sense the difference. When the difference is felt between these two items, the patient can test anything.

Hold-Sit-Test Method

This is the simplest procedure for self-testing allergies. Young patients love it; they often test secretly for their food, cookies, drinks, clothes, etc., using this method before the parents test them with NST.

Hold-Sit-Test Procedure

Step 1: Gather a sample holder (must be glass, not plastic, such as a thin glass jar, test tube, or a baby food jar with a lid), and samples of the suspected allergens. Each perishable item (e.g., liquid, food) should be placed inside the jar, then the lid should be closed tightly (plastic wrap between the jar and the lid helps prevent spills) so that the smell will not bother the patient. If the suspected allergen is a piece of fabric, toy, etc., it can be held in the hand. Severe allergens like pesticides, perfume, chemicals, or other toxic products should only be tested by adults, never by children.

Step 2: The patient holds the jar or small sample in the palm of the hand, touching the jar with the fingertips of the same hand for 15 to 30 minutes. If the patient is allergic to the sample, he/she will begin to feel uneasy when holding the allergen, giving rise to various unpleasant allergic symptoms, such as itching, sneezing, scratching, or some other symptom that was not present prior to holding the sample. The intensity of symptoms experienced is directly related to the severity of the allergy. Since the allergen is inside the sample holder when such uncomfortable sensations are felt, the allergen can be put away immediately and the patient can wash his/her hands to remove the energy of the allergen from the fingertips. This should stop the reaction immediately.

In this way, a patient can determine allergens and the degree of allergy easily without experiencing any real danger. Note: When patients with a history of anaphylaxis to a particular item are treated with NAET® for that item, this hold-sit-test method is used after completing the required NAET® treatments and before the patient begins to use the item again.

BENEFITS OF THE NAET®
DIAGNOSTIC APPROACH

It is amazing to find out how allergies can complicate existence and take the pleasure out of living. Most people will be amazed to find that allergies are the original cause of most common skin problems. Using the NAET® methods described in this chapter, readers can learn to test allergies and discover the cause of their skin problems.

If these simple testing skills can be learned and practiced by individuals with skin problems (as well as their families, guardians, caretakers, and doctors), it will not be long before they find out that most of their health problems (including eczema, acne, candidiasis and many other skin problems) have their roots in their daily diets, prescription medications, over-the-counter medications, enzymes, clothes, living environment, house cleaning chemicals, plastic accessories, cosmetics, soaps, detergents, hair shampoos and conditioners, hand soaps, moisturizers, body lotions, elastics, hand wipes, kitchen accessories, or products thought to be promoting health such as vitamins and supplements. If the person finds an item to be an allergen, then testing of other items should be performed until some non-allergic products can be found to use in daily life. Of course, the person who is allergic has the option to treat with NAET® and make the items non-allergic, or to avoid the items and never use them again.

When people learn to make a habit of testing everything with NAET® testing procedures for any possible hidden allergies, they will begin to uncover many of the hidden allergies in daily life. They may have been allergic to all of them for a long time, perhaps even since birth, but never bothered by them until their immune system went down due to some reason. Patients need to strengthen their immune system first, so that allergic reactions will be less bothersome. When people build up their immune system, their skin health also improves. Along the line, if patients can also eliminate the allergies by desensitizing with NAET® treatment, their skin problems will say good-bye forever.

CHAPTER 4

HOW ARE ALLERGY-RELATED SKIN DISORDERS TREATED?

Eliminating the Problem

OVERVIEW

*V*arious therapies and treatments are now available to help with allergy-related skin disorders. There is no one treatment or therapy made for everyone. General treatment approaches, used alone or in combination, now include:

- Western (conventional, allopathic) medicine approach
- Complementary and alternative medicine approach
- NAET® approach

This chapter will help patients understand these general treatment approaches, as well as the specific treatments available for:

- Eczema
- Acne
- Psoriasis
- Candidiasis
- Athlete's foot
- Baldness and Hair Loss

Patients need to investigate all available treatments. Please note, however, that all therapies and remedies described in this chapter are for educational purposes only. Diagnosis and treatment must still be managed by the patient's qualified doctor or health care professional.

WESTERN MEDICINE TREATMENT APPROACH

In general, Western medicine treatment approaches for allergy-related skin disorders may include:

- Avoidance of the offending allergen
- Symptomatic relief, using oral, injectable, or topical medications
- Antibiotics or antifungals, if a skin condition is from an infection, or if there is a secondary infection
- Phototherapy (ultraviolet radiation)
- Search for the root cause, and elimination of the cause if treatable

Each patient is unique, and should discuss the problem and treatment plan with his/her treating doctor.

COMPLEMENTARY AND ALTERNATIVE MEDICINE TREATMENT APPROACH

Overview

A number of alternative treatments have been used by practitioners and patients to find relief from eczema, acne, and other skin disorders, including:

- Avoidance of the offending allergen
- Acupuncture or acupressure treatments to help restore balance and reduce the discomfort of skin disorders
- Chiropractic treatment to remove the nerve impingement at the vertebral level and thus improve the nerve energy circulation to the affected area of the skin
- Herbal remedies (oral and topical) to cleanse and eliminate the internal toxins and to reduce symptoms
- Nutritional therapy and dietary supplements to provide the right support for vital organs and thus help the body heal itself
- Homeopathic remedies to help the overall condition and reduce symptoms
- Physical medicine (e.g., wet wraps or soaks) to help reduce symptoms of some conditions
- Lifestyle changes (e.g., exercise and hygiene) to help with normal circulation, prevention, and healing
- Mind-body medicine for stress reduction to help control flare-ups of conditions from stress, and to cope with the psychological complications from some skin conditions

General Herbal Remedies

Non-allergic topical creams or ointments can help relieve symptoms. (Note: Any cream or ointment applied to skin or affected area that causes burning, stinging, itching with increasing redness, hives, blisters, or swelling, should be washed off immediately and avoided until the allergy to that item is desensitized with NAET® treatment; so far NAET® is the only method that has been known to permanently eliminate allergies and sensitivities to the treated item.) Some of the herbal remedies known to assist in healing skin conditions include:

- Aloe vera - found in many topical creams and salves; helps heal the skin, and soothes symptoms such as itching, burning, and pain associated with eczema and other skin disorders
- Gotu kola - long used in Ayurvedic medicine, gotu kola helps treat rashes and thick skin, helps reduce itching and redness, and is useful in treating psoriasis
- Olive leaf - native to the Mediterranean region, olive leaf is a strong skin antiseptic, helping to fight infection and bacteria
- Red clover - a member of the pea family, red clover contains tocopherol, a powerful antioxidant that helps destroy toxins, to alleviate eczema and other chronic skin conditions
- Omega 3 fatty acids - people with skin conditions such as eczema often have fatty acid deficiencies, which may lead to the onset of the condition
- Zinc - this important mineral is crucial for proper fatty acid metabolism; a zinc deficiency could also lead to eczema and other skin disorders

Specific herbal remedy treatment options are mentioned for each condition later in this chapter. Some herbal remedies can cause unwanted side effects, or interact with conventional medications, so patients should discuss their treatment with a qualified health care professional.

General Nutritional Therapy

Healthy Diet

What is best for the body is best for the skin. (Note: Patients are encouraged to test their allergies using NAET® testing methods for anything that will be ingested.) A healthy, balanced diet with plenty of fruits and vegetables can be highly beneficial (after clearing the allergies with NAET® treatment for Vitamin C, fruits, and vegetables). When patients maintain adequate nutrition, the body tends to heal on its own, since it is provided with the right nutritional support to its vital organs. Many people now take vitamins, enzymes, and mineral supplements to ensure adequate nutritional intake, since many of today's foods have lost important nutrients due to canning, freezing, and other processing methods.

People with skin disorders are usually deficient in certain vitamins (Vitamins A, D, B-complex, and E), minerals (calcium, magnesium, zinc), and essential fatty acids (omega-3 and omega-6). Fatty acids taken orally help moisturize the skin naturally. If a person is allergic to fatty acids or fats, one of the symptoms is dry skin. Patients should make a routine of taking adequate non-allergic multivitamin/mineral supplements daily to maintain an adequate supply of nutrients. In addition to the daily vitamin-mineral formula, patients may consider taking an extra dose (RDA value) of calcium, Vitamin A, Vitamin D, and Vitamin B-complex. Drinking an adequate amount of fluids throughout the day is also important, to help eliminate toxins.

(Note: Supplements can also trigger itching, acne, eczema and other skin problems in many patients. Taking too many kinds of supplements at one time can result in interaction with each other and producing symptoms of excess. Patients are encouraged to use the NAET® QRT methods described in Chapter 3 to determine conditions of deficiency and/or excess from the supplements they take.)

Grape seed oil contains good fatty acids, and has many other health benefits. It is mild, so in allergic individuals it is less likely to cause a reaction compared with other fats and oils. Also, it does not have any strong taste or smell; most people including children may like the taste. Taking grape seed oil internally promotes healing from inside by assisting the clearance of any possible inflammation. Grape seed oil is known to have many essential vitamins (A, C, D, E, and beta carotene), antioxidants including proanthocyanidin, and fatty acids (omega-3, omega-6, and omega-9).

Nutrients to strengthen meridians. According or Oriental medicine, essential nutrients can strengthen acupuncture/energy meridians. For example:

Meridian. . . . . Essential nutrients to strengthen the meridian

Lung (Lu) . . . . Vitamins A, B-complex (especially B2), and C; proteins; bioflavonoids; essential fatty acids; cinnamon, onions, garlic, citrus fruits, green peppers, black peppers, rice; clear water

Large Intestine (LI). . . . Vitamins A, B1, C, D, E; wheat, wheat bran, oat bran, yogurt, roughage

Stomach (St) . . . . Vitamin B-complex (especially B12, B6, B3, and folic acid)

Spleen (Sp) . . . . Vitamins A and C; calcium, chromium; bioflavinoids, rutin, hesparin; protein;

berries, asparagus, hawthorn berries, or-
anges, root vegetables, sugar

Heart (Ht) . . . . Vitamins B-complex, C, and E; calcium,
selenium, potassium, sodium, iron; es-
sential fatty acids

Small Intestine (SI). . . . Vitamins B-complex, D, and E; essential
fatty acids; acidophilus, yogurt, fibers,
wheat germ, whole grains

Urinary Bladder (UB). . Vitamins A, B-complex (especially B1),
C, and E; calcium, trace minerals; amino
acids

Kidney (Ki). . . . . Vitamins A, B-complex, and E; sodium
chloride (table salt), trace minerals, cal-
cium, iron; essential fatty acids, amino
acids

Pericardium (Pc) . . . . . . Vitamins C and E; chromium, manga-
nese, trace minerals; lotus seed

Triple Warmer (TW) . . . Vitamin C; iodine, trace minerals, calcium, fluoride, zinc; vanadium; radish,
onion; water

Gall Bladder (GB). . . . . Vitamin A; calcium; linoleic acids and
oleic acids (e.g., in pine nuts, olive oil);
lemon

Liver (Liv). . . . . Vitamins A and F; trace minerals; beets,
green vegetables

Topical Application of Nutritional Supplements

Vitamin E is also beneficial as a topical application on skin affected by eczema or acne, since Vitamin E promotes healing. Grape seed oil is a preferred cosmetic ingredient for damaged and stressed tissues; its regenerative and restructuring qualities promote better skin hydration. When applied topically, it supports the cell membranes and can help skin retain the normal structure of epithelium cells and nerve cells.

Maintaining Alkalinity

Keeping the body slightly on the alkaline side (7.2 to 7.4 pH) can help reduce inflammation and itching due to eczema and other skin conditions. (Note: NAET® treatments for acid and base can help maintain the body's alkalinity.) Eating lots of non-allergic cooked or uncooked vegetables, drinking vegetable juices, barley green juice, liquid minerals, and alkalinized water on a daily basis can help. However, patients with eczema should avoid eating raw vegetables. Some of this author's patients have reported that drinking Xango® juice (after clearing the allergy to this item, if any) before meals has been helpful in reducing itching, dry skin, and eczema while going through NAET® treatments.

Lifestyle Changes

Exercise

Regular, mild, exercise is important to maintain the normal circulation needed to eliminate toxins produced inside the body. Gentle yoga exercises are ideal for patients suffering from eczema or other skin disorders.

Hygiene

Practicing better hygiene is essential with all skin conditions. (Note: Since some people are allergic to city water and tap water, patients should use NAET® NST described in Chapter 3 to locate a non-allergic water. Patients who are allergic to tap water should find a non-allergic bottled water for cleaning, bathing, and drinking until the allergy to tap water is cleared with NAET® treatment. Also, patients should check for allergy to any soap or product used on the skin, as well as towels used to dry the skin, and treat with NAET® to desensitize any allergies to those products.)

Patients should wash the affected area with a mild soap, rinse clean with water, and dry the skin with a soft cloth. Then patients should apply a non-allergic astringent (Sea Breeze®, witch hazel, etc.). Witch hazel is a gentle astringent with anti-inflammatory and healing properties. It helps to tighten pores and remove excess oil. To complete the routine, patients should apply a good, non-allergic moisturizer. Patients should follow this procedure three times daily until the skin condition heals.

Mind-Body Medicine: Addressing Stress and Emotions

Eczema, acne, and other common skin disorders can flare up when a person is under stress. Therefore, patients should learn how to recognize and cope with stress. It is essential to learn good relaxation techniques, and practice them regularly, to reduce stress.

Patients with eczema have significantly high levels of anxiety, and may have problems in dealing with anger and hostility. (Note: NAET® emotional balancing techniques can go to the root of the problems and help eliminate them. After eliminating core problems, patients may be better able to handle the psychological complications of their skin condition. Psychological counseling, group therapy, and relaxation techniques such as meditation and yoga work better after patients receive a few NAET® emotional balancing treatments with a well qualified NAET® Specialist.)

Stress includes external and internal stressors. External stressors are those that compromise the skin's ability to heal: sudden weather changes, exposure to dust, pollen, new fabric, formaldehyde, etc. Internal stressors are internalized emotions, such as anxiety, fear, low self-esteem, depression, frustration, etc. Emotional stressors can trigger chemical reactions inside the body that can result in eczema flare-ups and other skin irritations.

To combat external stressors, patients should find out the external triggers and avoid them. For example, changing activities to reduce daily stress can be helpful.

To manage internal stressors, patients should practice mild mind-calming exercises (such as meditation or yoga), drink plenty of water, and be well rested. Patients may want to maintain a checklist of "Things That Calm" in stressful times; calming activities might include reading a book, resting, listening to music, taking a walk, going to a movie, etc.

Relaxation Techniques
Practicing relaxation techniques can improve health in many ways. While stress causes the heart rate and blood pressure to increase, relaxation causes the heart rate and blood pressure to decrease. While stress often causes breathing to be fast and shallow, relaxation helps breathing to slow down and deepen. Together, improved heart rate and breathing improve the blood circulation to the peripheral tissues and muscle groups, enabling more oxygen and nutrients to reach the muscle tissue, which helps reduce overall tension, restlessness, irritability, anger, frustration, and desire for itching. Relaxation also promotes mental clarity, concentration, sleep, and healing of eczema.

Patients can learn and practice relaxation techniques on their own or with a group. Many resources are now available to learn relaxation techniques, including "how to" books, audio programs, video programs, and instruction from health care professionals. While some patients may prefer to learn and practice on their own, others may want to join a class. (Note: Some classes use aromatherapy or incense, which may cause allergic symptoms in sensitive people.)

Relaxation techniques usually involve an increased awareness of the body and a process that refocuses attention to something calming. It does not matter which technique is used; what matters is that relaxation is practiced regularly. Some simple but very effective relaxation techniques include autogenic relaxation, progressive muscle relaxation, and visualization.

Autogenic relaxation. "Autogenic" means "generated from within the person". In autogenic relaxation, the person uses both visual imagery and body awareness to reduce stress. The person repeats words or chants (a selected religious stanza, mantra, short devotional song, etc.) in the mind. Repetitions can be measured by time (e.g. for 30 minutes) or by number of repetitions (e.g., 100 times). It is important to keep track of progress (time elapsed or number of repetitions completed) during each session. This helps the person stay motivated to reach the goal, rather than becoming distracted from the relaxation process.

The idea is to focus the mind on something other than itching and scratching. After the relaxation technique is practiced, the person may experience an overall calmness: the mind is calm and relaxed, the nerves and muscles are relaxed, and the body functions are running smoothly. In this state, the person may either fall asleep peacefully, or resume daily activities without thinking about itching.

Progressive muscle relaxation. In this technique, the person focuses on one muscle group at a time, slowly tensing and then relaxing one muscle group before moving onto the next. This helps the mind focus on the difference between muscle tension and relaxation, and the person becomes more aware of physical sensations. One may choose to start with the muscles in the toes, then the feet, then the lower legs, and so on, progressively moving up to the muscles in the neck and head. Or, one can begin from the top of the head and work down towards the toes. Muscles in each group should be tensed for at least five seconds, then relaxed for 30 seconds; this cycle should be repeated at least ten times in each muscle group. This entire process may take 30 minutes or longer, depending on the person's preference, needs, and time available.

Visualization. This technique involves using mental images to take a visual journey in the mind. Before starting this process, the person may want to find a comfortable place, away from noises and people (e.g., without the dog barking, children crying, telephone ringing nonstop, etc.). The person may either sit up or lay down on a comfortable surface, and any tight clothing should be comfortably loosened. Then, closing the eyes, the person forms mental images to take a visual journey to wherever he/she would like to go. This mental journey could be to a sandy and mildly sunny warm beach; a gentle and soothing waterfall; a whispering Amazon rain forest; a peaceful valley; a golf course; a peaceful calming place; etc. It helps to engage as many senses as possible, including smells, sights, sounds, and textures. For example, if the person imagines relaxing at the beach, it helps to think about the fragrance of the ocean and sand, the sparkling sun on the crystal blue water, the warmth of the sun, the crackling sound of the crashing waves, the smoothness of the grainy sand under bare feet, the caressing soft breeze against the cheeks, etc. This author teaches patients to visualize the 12 acupuncture meridians, and to imagine tracing them a few times, from the lung meridian to the end of liver meridian. Tracing the meridians provides another benefit: it can remove accumulated imbalances in the meridians, and help nerve energy move freely and smoothly, bringing the body into a homeostatic (balanced) state. According to Oriental medical principles, a body with free flowing nerve energy is in a perfect balance – a blissful state. In that state, the body will not experience any allergy or disease. Meridian balancing procedures done visually in this way, or physically with acupuncture or acupressure, can produce similar results.

Other relaxation techniques. Yoga, Tai chi, music, exercise, meditation, and hypnosis are also beneficial in reducing stress. Physical medicine (e.g., soaks or wet wraps) can also help. Epsom salt soaking of the whole body in lukewarm/tepid water, or a cold shower, may help with itching and hives, while reducing stress and nervousness. (Note: If the person is allergic to cold water, warm water is okay, but very hot water should be avoided.) Cold water or wet wraps with cold towels may reduce itching and pain if applied to the affected area. Patients should follow the advice of their doctor or health care professional.

NAET®
TREATMENT APPROACH

Overview

According to NAET® theory, most skin disorders (especially eczema) develop from some form of allergy (see Chapter 2). Without eliminating the hypersensitivities, intolerances, and allergies to the foods consumed and the products contacted on a daily basis, patients are not likely to eliminate their skin problems. All of the therapies and remedies currently available may help control symptoms for awhile, but the moment a person stops the therapies or remedies, symptoms are likely to return. This author and many patients personally experienced this struggle for many years until the allergies were eliminated through NAET®, as described in the case studies throughout this book. Though it may seem tedious to be treated with NAET® for all known allergens, one by one, it is worth it. When the allergies are gone, patients have the freedom to return to normal living.

Statistics show that 80%-90% of allergic patients who receive proper NAET® treatments, and who cooperate with the doctor, are either entirely relieved of eczema and other skin conditions, or are satisfactorily improved. NAET® treatment can provide satisfying results if done properly. NAET® Specialists from around the world can be found via the "doctor locator" at www.naet.com; these health care providers have received special training in NAET®, and some have also received special training in management of skin disorders.

Treatment with NAET® is focused on:

- **NAET® desensitization treatments for all known allergens.** The NAET® Specialist uses NAET® diagnostic methods (see Chapter 3) to test NAET® Basic allergens and Classic allergens, then desensitizes the patient for each allergen in the given order. It is extremely important to follow the order of treatments, because the contents of the first allergen mixtures overlap with the contents of many other allergen mixtures that follow in the given order. Often desensitization for NAET® Basic allergens helps to clear allergies to the remaining Classic allergens without further treatments. So, soon after treating for the Basic allergens, the NAET® Specialist can begin testing and treating by priority, or for other necessary combinations.

- **NAET® self-balancing with acupressure.** Patients are encouraged to self-balance using specific acupressure points. By massaging these points once or twice a day as a routine, patients can help prevent itching and other discomforts. Patients who experience any itching, hives, edema, acne, eczema, or other allergy-related symptoms can follow acute care self-balancing procedures every ten minutes until the acute problem is relieved. Resuscitation points can be used in cases of emergency. Patients should also drink two glasses of non-allergic water (testing the water first via NST) immediately, and then drink four glasses of non-allergic water daily, since energy flows well in a well-hydrated body.

- **Supportive therapies.** Any of the Western medicine or complementary and alternative therapies mentioned for the specific condition can be used to help reduce allergy-based symptoms while going through initial NAET® treatments. After most of the allergens (Basic, Classic, and others by priority) are desensitized with NAET® treatment, patients usually experience great relief from the original problem and no longer need these supportive therapies.

In addition, avoidance helps prevent flare-ups until an allergen is desensitized with NAET® treatment. Patients and their loved ones need to determine what triggers symptoms (see Chapter 2), so that these triggers can be avoided. Patients are also encouraged to take time to read, learn, and master the self-testing methods described in Chapter 3, to detect the triggers at home and strictly avoid them until receiving appropriate help. It takes practice to do these self-tests appropriately, but patients and loved ones should not become discouraged. Everyone needs to practice for many hours before the NST technique starts working to deliver accurate results.

NAET® Desensitization Treatments

Most people who suffer from skin problems find that their symptoms are controlled or eliminated when they successfully complete NAET® treatment for the Basic and Classic groups of allergens. While some people with mild or moderate skin problems may show marked improvements after completing only a few of the Basic allergens, it is to their advantage to complete treatment for all of the Basic and Classic allergens, so that they have an ample selection of foods to eat without having to worry about reactions. People with severe health problems or skin problems may need even more treatments before they can experience complete freedom from their symptoms.

NAET® Basic Allergens
(in preferred order of treatment)

1. BBF (Brain body balance formula)
2. Egg mix (animal protein, egg white, egg yolk, chicken)
3. Calcium mix (cow milk, goat milk, different types of calcium)
4. Vitamin C mix

5. Vitamin B-complex
6. Sugar mix (children with eczema may develop diabetes at later years)
7. Iron mix
8. Vitamin A mix
9. Minerals, trace minerals (water, city water)
10. Salt mix
11. Grains (wheat, rice, corn, oat, rye, millet)
12. Yeast mix, yogurt, whey
13. Stomach acid [acidity]
14. Digestive enzymes or base [alkalinity]
15. Hormones (estrogen, progesterone, testosterone)
16. Organ mix (individual organs can be treated here)
17. RNA and DNA (skin problems, especially eczema cases, may need to check each and every item treated in combination with DNA, since most allergies and eczema cases are genetic in nature)

NAET® Classic Allergens

The NAET® Classic allergens include the NAET® Basic allergen groups (listed above), and several other major allergen groups (listed below). NAET® treatments should preferably be given in the order listed. Each item should also be checked in combination with DNA. Approximately 80% of a patient's allergic reactions towards substances will diminish if that patient clears 100% on all of the Classic allergens.

1. Hypothalamus
2. Hypothalamus + DNA
3. Heat
4. Cold
5. Humidity
6. Dryness
7. Dampness
8. Sympathetic nerves
9. Parasympathetic nerves

10. Artificial sweeteners
11. Coffee, chocolate, caffeine
12. Spice mix 1 and 2
13. Vegetable fat, animal fat
14. Nut mix 1 and 2
15. Fish and shell fish
16. Amino acids 1 and 2
17. Filaggrin (a special protein for the skin)
18. Whiten-all
19. Turkey / serotonin
20. Fluoride
21. Gum mix
22. Dried bean mix
23. Alcohol
24. Gelatin
25. Vitamin D
26. Vitamin E
27. Vitamin F (fatty acids)
28. Vitamin T (thymus)
29. Individual amino acids
30. Chromosome mix
31. Food coloring / food additives
32. Starch mix (carbohydrates)
33. Nightshade vegetables / vegetable mix
34. Virus mix
35. Bacteria mix
36. Parasites
37. Chemicals (soap, detergent, etc.)
38. Pollens
39. Grasses / weeds
40. Formaldehyde
41. Latex / plastics
42. Crude oil / synthetic materials, etc.
43. Animal epithelial /dander
44. Smoking / nicotine
45. Dust / dust mites

46. Perfume mix / flowers
47. Immunizations / vaccinations / drugs
48. Body parts or tissues (a particular part of the body that is involved with the disease process, e.g., lung, liver, hypothalamus, thyroid, adrenals, pituitary, knee, elbow)
49. Neurotransmitters
50. Pesticides
51. Heavy metals

Other Allergens

- After-shave lotion, razor blades
- Animals, their epithelial and dander
- Bed, bed linen, bed sheet, comforter, and blanket
- Books, papers, and magazines
- Carpets and drapes
- Ceramic cups and tiles on the floor
- Chemicals, soap, and detergents
- Child's schoolwork materials
- Clothing, bath towels and other fabrics
- Colored clothes (people can be allergic to different colors)
- Coloring books
- Computer screen, keyboard, desk, and chair
- Cooking dishes and utensils
- Dishwashing soaps and scrubbers
- Drinks, drinking water, and tap water
- Eating utensils (e.g., plates, spoons, fork)
- Fruits and vegetables
- Nightgowns, pajamas
- Grains and breads
- Hair shampoo, hair conditioner, and body lotions
- Housecleaning products
- Latex gloves and office products
- Leaves, weeds, grass, and flowers
- Lipstick and other cosmetics
- Oils, and other food items
- Newspaper and ink

- Pens, pencils, and writing paper
- Pillows and pillow cases
- Salts and sugars
- Telephones
- Toothbrush, toothpaste, mouthwash, and dental floss
- Toothpick, Q-tips, other hygienic materials
- Toys and stuffed animals
- Vitamins and drugs
- Work materials

Each NAET® desensitization treatment begins with NAET® NST/QRT (see Chapter 3), then a process that consists of stimulating certain specific points on the acupuncture meridians while holding the allergen being desensitized (see Figure 4-1). This process produces the necessary immune mediators (like antidotes) to neutralize the adverse reaction coming from the allergen held in the hand, resulting in a totally new, permanent, and irreversible response to the allergen.

Each treatment is followed by a 25-hour avoidance period for the allergen being treated. (People tend to fall out of treatments when the allergens are not avoided for 25 hours. In some cases, this author has observed that a patient may need to avoid the treated food allergen for 30 hours or more. This may be due to the fact that the individual has a lower level immune system, probably due to chronic illnesses, or has a stronger allergy to that item.) After completing the desensitization and 25-hour avoidance period, each item from the treated group should be tested individually again, to be certain that the treatment for each individual ingredient from the group has been completed. Some highly sensitive individuals may need repeated treatments on individual ingredients of the mixes to satisfactorily complete the desensitization. For example, though a person may have cleared the "egg mix" group, that person may need additional treatments for one or more of the individual ingredients in that mix, such as egg white, egg yolk, tetracycline, or feathers. The NAET® Specialist will give each patient information on the specific item that needs to be desensitized. A full

NAET® treatment program may require as few as 10 office visits, or as many as 100 or more office visits, depending on the patient's immune system, the severity of the patient's condition, the patient's age, and the patient's willingness and ability to follow the after-treatment instructions.

While patients go through the NAET® treatment program, they should practice NAET® QRT (see Chapter 3) at home so that by the time the NAET® treatment is completed for the necessary allergen groups, they will be confident in self-testing and self-screening before exposing themselves to new substances. This is the only way that patients will prevent future incidents of eczema, acne, itching, and any other problems: by learning to take charge of their health.

Note: People who successfully complete NAET® treatment for a particular food product should be aware that the contents and food additives in these products may change with each batch or new purchase. For example: a patient may have been treated for milk on January 8, 2006 and the facial acne disappeared the next day. But that patient may have bought a new carton of milk a few days later, drank that milk, then broke out in a whole-body rash on June 12, 2006. If that patient had used NST before purchasing or drinking the new milk, he/she would have discovered a sensitivity to that new milk, even though treatment was successful for another milk batch on January 8th. The new milk may have had several different ingredients for which that patient was not treated. For example, the cow that secreted the new milk may have been fed some products that were allergens for this patient, and the essence of the allergen was in the milk, thus causing a reaction; or, this milk may have processed slightly differently; or, the container may have been contaminated with pesticides, bacteria, or something else. To avoid unexpected surprises, patients must learn to test everything before use.

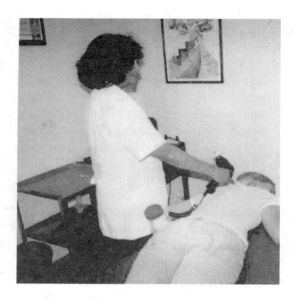

*Figure 4-1. NAET®
treatment.*

NAET® Rotation Diet

Patients are advised to maintain a food diary and bring it to the NAET® Specialist on each visit. If the patient has an allergic reaction while going through the treatment program, the trigger can be traced more easily and then treated, thus preventing further pain.

The NAET® rotation diet refers to eating non-allergic foods in a certain order. After patients have cleared their allergy to the NAET® Basic allergens, foods from the allergy-free list are consumed in a pre-selected order, to help the body eliminate toxins that had accumulated prior to the Basic allergen treatments. This rotation diet also helps patients maintain better health with less itching and pain. To determine the non-allergic items, the NAET® Specialist uses NAET® NST/QRT as described in Chapter 3. Every meal is then selected from a non-reactive list according to the priority. This prevents overload of the particular food in the body, and reduces unwanted allergic reactions. As time goes on, the patient will have plenty of foods to eat without triggering allergic symptoms.

NAET® Treatment by Priority

After successfully completing NAET® treatment for the Basic allergens, the NAET® Specialist will evaluate the patient's progress. If needed, additional treatment will be given by priority to help with any immediate health problem, such as treating the allergen that will help with that patient's eczema, acne, dry skin, itching, athlete's foot, yeast problem, dandruff, etc. After the Basic allergens, the rest of the NAET® Classic allergen groups can be rearranged to help with the immediate problem. This is called "treatment by priority". For example:

- If the patient's major complaint was "hand eczema," after completing treatment for the Basic allergens, if the hand eczema is still not under control, the NAET® Specialist will begin treating specific allergens related to triggering that condition, such as the patient's new hand lotion, latex gloves, the new hand soap, dish scrubber in the kitchen, the portable phone received as a gift, hot water, humidity, etc.

- If the patient had suffered from facial acne for the last two months, soon after the patient completes treatment for the Basic allergens, the NAET® Specialist will treat for the new wash cloth, the face cream, the new make-up, the patient's favorite salad dressing that is eaten daily for the last two months, etc.

All individual treatments work better after the patient successfully clears allergies to essential nutrients, i.e., the NAET® Basic allergens. Through 25 years of experience in this field, this author has observed that when patients receive NAET® "treatment by priority" without having completed treatment for the Basic allergens, these patients require many more treatments (perhaps even hundreds of treatments) to receive the same benefit available from completing as few as 20 treatments (i.e., completing treatment for the Basic allergens in preferred order, then receiving "treatment by priority").

If patients see their NAET® Specialist for any acute allergic reaction (itching, hives, rashes, painful acne, etc.), if the NAET® Specialist is confident in treating the acute symptom, the allergen or group of allergens may be treated out of the preferred order. If the practitioner is not experienced or confident to treat the acute problem, perhaps if it is a whole-body rash with hives, accompanied by restlessness and fever (probably a severe allergic reaction to a food), patients should call for emergency help (such as 911 in United States). When the acute symptom is resolved, patients can begin treatment for the first allergen in the Basics group. When done properly, NAET® treatments can give patients quick and lasting relief. If not done properly, patients may not receive the expected results. After completing treatment for the Basic allergen groups, patients who do not see any improvement in their condition should discuss and evaluate this with their practitioner.

NAET® Self-Balancing With Acupressure

Patients are encouraged to perform self-balancing procedures to help control symptoms while going through NAET® desensitization treatments. Information and illustrations for a few important acupressure points, including NAET® general balancing points, resuscitation points, and points for specific conditions, are provided in the following pages. These points and techniques, when used properly according to the accompanying instructions, might help to reduce or control allergic symptoms. These balancing techniques are safe to use on people at any age and in any condition.

When one maintains energy in a balanced state, the body may not experience any illness or adverse reactions. Many patients have reported that they were able to keep their allergic reactions under control simply through regular self-balancing. Some have reported a reduction in their other allergy-related health conditions as well. Note: These are only energy balancing techniques,

and should not be confused with actual NAET® treatment procedures performed by a trained NAET® Specialist. These balancing
techniques will not replace the need for a trained NAET® Specialist.

General Self-Balancing Points

Patients may use the general balancing points shown in Figure
4-2 while going through treatments with a NAET® Specialist. This
will help patients finish the NAET® treatments more quickly and
easily. The general self-balancing procedure is as follows.

Step 1: Become familiar with the location of each balancing
point. (Some points are on both sides of the body.)

Step 2: Cycle through each essential point in the order shown.
Using the pads of the fingers, gently massage each point in a clockwise direction for 1 minute (15 seconds if using a point stimulator). This cycle can be done 1-2 times a day.

Patients need not be sick to benefit from balancing the body.
These techniques can be practiced with or without NAET® treatments, any time a person feels out of balance. How do people
know if their body is out of balance? A normally health person
who is slightly out of balance may not feel sick, but may not feel
quite right. Perhaps that person feels tired, sleepy in the afternoon,
unmotivation to do normal work activities, or mild general itching on the body or foot etc., but that person cannot find a definite
reason for such "out of sorts" feeling. A mild allergy to something
that the person ate, drank or touched may be causing some minor
energy disturbance in the meridians. If that person can immediately balance the body using these acupressure points, the energy
blockage can be cleared from the meridians, and that person will
feel normal in minutes.

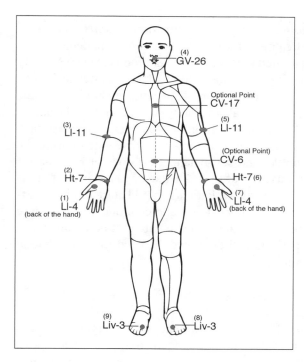

Figure 4-2.
Acupressure points
for general
self-balancing.

Location of essential points:

LI-4: On the back of the hand, it is midway between the long bones of the thumb and index finger, approximately 1 inch above the web

Ht-7: On the inside of the wrist, it is on the medial side (same side as 5th finger) on the wrist crease

LI-11: When the elbow is flexed, it is at the outside end of the elbow crease

GV-26: Below the nose, it is just above the midpoint of the vertical groove in the upper lip area

Liv-3: Near the toes, it is in the soft area between where the 1st and 2nd long bones in the foot end

Location of additional points:

CV-17: On the midline of the breastbone, it is between the nipples, level with the 4th space between the ribs

CV-6: On the midline of the abdomen, it is 2 finger breadths below the "belly button"

Self-balancing for daily foods and supplements. After successful NAET® treatment for the Basic allergens, patients should begin collecting a small portion of different foods consumed daily at each meal in a glass container, and self-balance after each meal using the points shown in Figure 4-2. Patients should continue self-balancing for each meal separately for one month. Then, patients should collect a small portion of each item (from breakfast, lunch, dinner, and whatever else they may have eaten during the day) in a glass bottle, and self-balance just once at bedtime for this entire day's mixture; after this balancing, the patient puts the day's single sample away. Patients should start a new collection of food samples on the next day, and continue this procedure for a year. The benefits of this approach are that no avoidance is necessary, and patients will eliminate the need for NAET® food combination treatments.

Acute Care

Resuscitation. If a person experiences an emergency — sudden symptoms such as fainting, sudden loss of consciousness, cardiac arrhythmia, heart attack, stroke, sudden loss of energy, hypoglycemia, heat stroke, sudden pain in the lower back, general lower backache, breathing problem due to allergic reactions, mental confusion, mental irritability, anger, uncontrollable rage, exercise-induced anaphylaxis, anaphylactic reactions to allergens, sudden breathing problem due to any cause, sudden itching, severe itching, etc. — any of the resuscitation points shown in Figure 4-3 can help until qualified professional help arrives. The acupressure resuscitation procedure is simple.

Step 1: At the beginning of the problem, massage or stimulate any of the points gently but firmly, in a clockwise direction, for 30-60 seconds.

People who want to wake up from sleeping while driving, or recover from sudden loss of energy, can massage gently on the

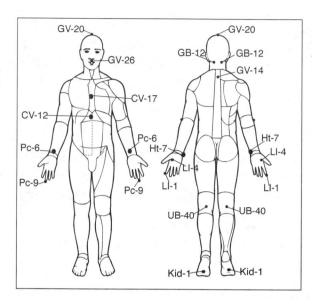

Figure 4-3.
Acupressure points for resuscitation.

GV-26: Below the nose, a little above the midpoint of the vertical groove in the upper lip area

CV-17: On the midline of the breastbone, between the nipples, level with the 4th space between ribs

CV-12: On the midline of the abdomen, 3.75 inches above the belly button

Pc-6: Three finger-breadths above the wrist crease on the palmar side

Pc-9: On the center of the tip of the middle finger

GB-12: On the underside of the skull where the large muscle (sternocleidomastoid, or "SCM") is attached

GV-14: Below the 7th cervical vertebra, approximately at the level of the shoulders

Ht-7: On the inside of the wrist, it is on the medial side (same side as 5th finger) on the wrist crease

LI-4: On the back of the hand, it is midway between the long bones of the thumb and index finger, approximately 1 inch above the web

LI-1: On the index finger (thumb side), at the corner of the fingernail

UB-40: In the middle of the crease on the back of the knee, in the soft spot between tendons

Kid-1: On the sole near the end of the long bones of the foot, in the space that appears when the foot is flexed downward

GV-26 point (below the nose). For example, if a person is driving and suddenly feels loss of energy or sensation of fainting, that person should immediately massage this point. That person's energy will begin to circulate faster and a fainting episode may be prevented.

For more information on revival techniques, refer to *"Acupuncture: A Comprehensive Text"*, or *"Living Pain Free with Acupressure"* (see Bibliography).

Specific conditions. If a person is having an acute skin problem, the treating doctor should be consulted. Until professional help arrives, a person may be able to help bring symptoms under control using acupressure. The acupressure procedure for specific acute conditions is as follows.

Step 1: Use the general body balancing procedure described above (with points shown in Figure 4-2).

Step 2: Use acupressure on the points specific to the patient's condition. (Acupressure points for eczema, hives, acne, psoriasis, candidiasis, athlete's foot, and hair loss are illustrated under the treatment section for each of these conditions, later in this chapter.) Note: acupressure methods vary somewhat, depending on the patient's goal:

- For more energy (if exhausted or weak, e.g., with an infection)
  - o Using the pads of the fingers, gently tap, or massage points in clockwise direction; or, use a point stimulator
  - o 30 seconds on each point (15 seconds if using a point stimulator)
  - o 1-2 times a day
- For relief from too much energy (e.g., feeling overstimulated from too much itching)

- o Using the pads of the fingers, gently massage points in a counter-clockwise direction; or, use a point stimulator
- o 1-3 minutes on each point (30 seconds if using a point stimulator)
- o 2-4 times a day
- For pain relief
  - o Using the pads of the fingers, gently massage points in a counter-clockwise direction; or, use a point stimulator
  - o 1 minute on each point (30 seconds if using a point stimulator)
  - o Every 5-10 minutes, 6-10 times or until pain is relieved

It is also helpful to drink two glasses of non-allergic water (test the water via NST) immediately, and then drink four tall glasses of non-allergic water daily. Energy flows well in a well-hydrated body. (There is a simple way to find out a person's total daily water requirement, as measured in ounces. First, determine the person's weight in pounds, then divide it by 2. For example, if a person weighs 120 pounds, 120/2=60, so that person's daily water requirement is 60 ounces. This translates to 7.5 cups/day (1 cup = 8 ounces, 60/8=7.5).

Some patients can experience pain, emotional release, or increased itching during an acupressure session. If the patient has an emotional blockage, for best results it should be isolated and treated with NAET®. If the patient has itching or pain during an acupressure session, the cycle of acupressure point treatment should be repeated; often this will stop the itching or pain.

Supportive Therapies and the NAET® Rice-Detox Diet

Many supportive therapies are available. General approaches (Western and complementary) as well as specific treatments for common skin disorders are described in this chapter.

In addition, the NAET® Rice-Detox Diet may be helpful.

The NAET® Rice-Detox Diet
Before using this recipe, patients should ensure that they are not allergic to any of these ingredients. The health benefits of the ingredients in this recipe include:

- Clearing neurotoxins from the brain and nervous system (coriander)
- Cleansing the sinuses, glands and lymphatic system (coriander seeds)
- Clearing the liver meridian and spleen meridian (coriander)
- Strengthening the spleen meridian (brown sugar)
- Strengthening the liver meridian (dandelion leaves)
- Cleansing and strengthening the lung meridian (cinnamon, lemon rind, and rice)
- Strengthening the heart and circulatory systems (pepper)
- Strengthening the stomach meridian (ginger root)
- Strengthening the gall bladder meridian (coconut oil)
- Strengthening the urinary bladder meridian (lemon leaves)
- Strengthening the kidney meridian (rock salt)
- Cleaning and strengthening the small intestine meridian, plus antibacterial properties (turmeric and cumin seed)
- Strengthening the large intestine meridian (pomegranate)
- Clearing toxins from the whole system (garlic, which is a natural antibacterial, antiparasitic, and antioxidant)

This author often prepares this rice recipe even now, because this spicy, delicious rice once saved her life! (See Preface.)

Recipe – Rice Detox

Ingredients (ensure all are non-allergic):

1 cup	Rice (uncooked)
8 cups	Water
2 tablespoons	Coriander powder
1 teaspoon	Coriander leaves (fresh, chopped)
1 teaspoon	Butter (fresh, clarified)
1 teaspoon	Coconut oil (fresh)
1 teaspoon	Herbal detox powder (recipe below)
To taste	Salt

Preparation:

Rinse the rice four times with clean water, cook well in eight cups of water, and drain when the rice is cooked well. Add coriander powder, three ounces of water and cook again under slow fire until the water is evaporated completely. Add rest of the ingredients, mix well and cover and keep it for 10 minutes before serving.

Recipe – Herbal Detox Powder

Ingredients (equal amounts of each):

Brown sugar	Lemon leaves
Cinnamon	Lemon rind
Coriander seeds	Pepper
Cumin seed	Pomegranate powder
Dandelion	Rock salt
Garlic powder	Turmeric
Ginger root powder	

Preparation:

Add equal amounts of each ingredient to a bowl, and grind into a fine powder.

TREATMENT FOR ECZEMA

Though eczema can be painful, it is not fatal or contagious (as long as it is not a symptom of some more serious disease or disorder). Eczema does not have harmful long-term effects, except for poor quality of life and the possibility of losing workdays. Today, many effective therapies are available to treat the different types of eczema. With proper treatment, most eczema can be controlled or cured.

Western Medicine Treatment

Currently there is no effective treatment for eczema/dermatitis using only conventional treatment. However, there are many ways to avoid the eczema triggers once detected, and to minimize the discomfort and distress from eczema. Conventional treatment may include:

- Lifestyle changes: avoiding anything that triggers symptoms, keeping fingernails short and avoiding scratching, protecting skin from irritants, trying to reduce stress, and keeping environment cool with stable temperature and humidity
- Anti-itch treatments: lotions, ointments, or tablets with a corticosteroid (e.g., hydrocortisone cream in a hypoallergenic base, or prednisone tablets); cream that contains tar compounds; lotions that lubricate or soften the skin; topical immunomodulators that are steroid-free (e.g., tacrolimus, ascomycin)
- Antihistamines may not be very effective but are sometimes given at night if sleeping is a problem
- Antibiotics (creams or pills) if there is secondary infection

- If the eczema is more severe, phototherapy (a type of treatment that uses light therapy) may be prescribed; if it is given with a medication, this symptomatic treatment is called photochemotherapy

Some doctors think that allergy shots, also called "allergen immunotherapy", may be helpful for patients with eczema (atopic dermatitis). Allergy shots, which are like vaccines for the offending allergens, work by injecting the allergen in increasing doses so that the body's immune system can develop immunity. The shots can help with allergies to pollens, dust mites, cockroaches, mold, pet dander, and stinging insects such as bees and wasps. But the shots do not work for everyone or for all allergies (e.g., they do not work for people with food allergies). Also, sometimes there are side effects. Allergy shots need to be given weekly for a few months, then monthly for up to five years.

Patients should discuss their treatment plan with their dermatologist.

Complementary and Alternative Treatment

Many complementary therapies are available to reduce the discomfort of eczema:

- Nutritional therapy and dietary supplements, such as essential fatty acids (Gamma-linolenic acid, or "GLA"), probiotics ("good" bacteria), sulfur, zinc, bromelain, and Vitamins A, C, and E; or topical cream with Vitamin B12
- Herbal remedies, such as evening primrose oil, lavender, burdock root, German chamomile, goldenrod, red clover, roman chamomile, stinging nettle, flavinoids, sarsaparilla, gotu kola; also, creams or salves with forchamomile, chickweed, marigold, licorice, witch hazel, peppermint/ menthol, or St. John's wort

- Homeopathic remedies, such as calendula, sulphur, urtica urens, rhus toxicodendron, antimonium crudum, apis mellifica
- Physical medicine, such as soaking the area in a bath containing rice starch
- Massage (only if the skin is not actively inflamed), to help reduce stress
- Exercise (only if the skin is not in the worst stage of symptoms), to help feel better emotionally
- Mind-body medicine, to help reduce anxiety and stress
- Lifestyle changes, such as avoiding known irritants, taking care of the skin, bathing with mild soap, minimizing scratching, and wearing gloves

Some of these treatments (especially some herbal remedies) could have side effects. It is important for patients to be treated by a qualified health care professional.

Lifestyle Changes

Avoiding known irritants. Too much heat and sweat can make the skin more irritated and itchy. Patients should try to avoid spending a lot of time in an extremely warm or cold atmosphere, or in activities that make them feel hot and sweaty. It helps to avoid contact with irritants that trigger itching or rash, such as household cleansers, soap, detergents, after-shave lotions, gasoline and other solvents, wool, and some synthetic fabrics.

Skin care. Dry skin is fairly common with eczema. Dry skin causes more itching and inflammation, so proper care should be taken to reduce these symptoms. Keeping the skin well moisturized is one of the best ways to reduce dryness.

Gentle bathing. Patients should bathe only with a small amount of mild soap. Water temperature should be cool or warm, not hot. Soaking in the tub for 15 to 20 minutes (in a non-allergic water) can be good for the skin, because the skin's outer layer can absorb water and become less dry. After the bath, a soft towel should be used to pat the skin dry without rubbing. Immediately after drying, a good moisturizer (such as one with grape seed oil, ensuring that it is non-allergic) should be applied to the skin.

Minimizing scratching. Scratching can break the skin. Patients (or parents of patients) should make a point to cut the patient's fingernails and toenails regularly, to a short length, then file the nails smooth. Patients may also wear cotton gloves or any other soft non-allergic gloves to prevent scratching. If the patient scratches and breaks the skin, bacteria can enter the body, which may lead to secondary infections by *Streptococcus* or *Staphylococcus* bacteria.

Wearing gloves. Since soaps or wetness can cause skin irritation, hands should only be washed when necessary, especially if there is eczema on the hands. Hands should be dried completely after washing. When work requires that hands be in water, patients should wear non-allergic vinyl or plastic gloves to help prevent irritation. Cotton gloves can be worn under plastic gloves to soak up sweat from the hands. (It helps to take occasional breaks by removing the gloves to prevent a buildup of sweat inside the gloves.) During the winter, patients should wear gloves to protect from the cold air and low humidity that can dry the skin, which can make eczema worse.

NAET® Treatment

NAET® treatment for eczema involves strengthening the immune system (treating with NAET® for Basic and Classic allergens), and avoiding and/or treating with NAET® for allergens commonly associated with eczema, which include:

- Ingestants: Proteins, fish, shell fish, nuts, milk products, wheat products, starches, fruits, corn, vegetable

and animal fats, food additives, sugar products, candy,
chocolate, chewing gums, prescription drugs, vitamin
supplements (especially Vitamin C products), herbs,
trace minerals, chromium, drinking water
- Contactants: Cosmetics, body lotions, soaps, detergents,
fabric softeners, fabrics, chemicals, carpets, pets, lactic
acid, sweat, city water, chlorinated water
- Inhalants: Perfume, tobacco smoke, chemicals
- Infectants: Parasites, infections
- Physical agents: Heat and humidity
- Psychogenic causes: Emotional stressors

In addition:

- Patients should avoid and/or treat with NAET® as needed
for stiff and tight clothing, particular when it contains
coarse wool products, polyester, or strong dyes. The
patient is usually the best judge of which fabric causes
itching.
- If the patient's skin is dry, in addition to using non-allergic lotions, NAET® treatment for dryness helps reduce
the dryness naturally.
- People have developed eczema from allergy to formaldehyde. The main source of formaldehyde exposure is
from the nametags of the ready-made clothes. Nametags
usually cause eczema on the skin surface where the tags
rub against upon wearing: lower back, mid-back (from
bra), back of the neck and sides of the thighs.
- Wearing non-allergic slippers and shoes can help prevent
foot ulcers and foot eczema.
- Many people are allergic to their own fingernails.
Scratching with the allergic nails worsens the existing
eczema. In these cases, patients should treat with NAET®
for their own fingernails.
- While going through the NAET® treatments, patients
may need some good supportive care (such as those

described in Western and complementary approaches, above) to keep symptoms under control.

- Patients may also use acupressure self-help as described earlier in this chapter; the points specific to eczema are shown in Figure 4-4.

Hives. For patients with hives, commonly seen allergens include: NAET® Basics and Classics, tomatoes, fish, shellfish, fruits, milk products, corn, salt, sugar, food additives, food colors, yeast, chocolate, fabrics, chemicals, cleansing chemicals, weeds, grasses, poison ivy, peaches, cashew nuts, onions, melons, peppers, and spices. Acupressure points specific to hives are shown in Figure 4-5.

Children With Eczema and Other Skin Problems

For children in particular, the itchiness of eczema can be very distressing. There are many methods of reducing the itchiness of the skin and minimizing the damage from scratching. Their fingernails and toenails should be kept short and smooth. Their symptom triggers should be tested, and either strictly avoided or treated with NAET®. Cotton clothing and bedding will help keep the skin cool and allow it to breathe (if the child is not allergic to cotton). Synthetic fabrics and wool should be avoided, since they can irritate the skin. Itchy skin can also be reduced by using a non-biological washing powder, and avoiding use of fabric softeners.

Children should also be desensitized with NAET® for common triggers, such as dust, dust mites, mattresses, bed, night-wear, skin creams, soaps, and detergents used on the bed linens. Parents should continue to follow the tips in this section even after the child's skin has healed, to prevent future flare-ups.

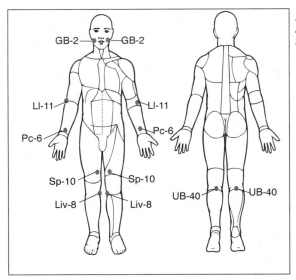

Figure 4-4.
Acupressure points
for ECZEMA.

Point locations:

GB-2:   Between the ear and the top of the jawbone

LI-11:   When the elbow is flexed, it is at the outside end of the
elbow crease

Pc-6:   Three finger breadths above the wrist crease on the
palmar side

Sp-10:   When the knee is flexed, 3 finger-breadths above the
top edge of the patella, on the inside of the thigh; feel
for pain or tenderness at the spot

Liv-8:   On the inside of the knee joint, behind the top edge of
the tibia (which is the large long bone in the bottom part
of the leg)

UB-40:   In the middle of the crease on the back of the knee, in
the soft spot between tendons

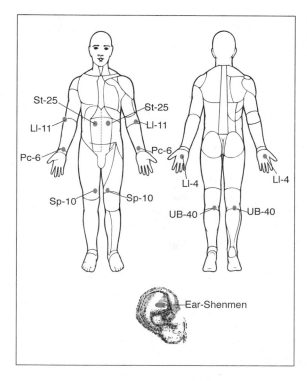

Figure 4-5.
Acupressure
points for HIVES.

Point locations:

Ear-Shenmen: *At the outside edge of the V-shaped depres-*
sion that is near the top of the ear

St-25: *Four finger-breadths to the side of the center of the*
belly button

LI-11: *When the elbow is flexed, it is at the outside end of*
the elbow crease

Pc 6: *Three finger breadths above the wrist crease on the*
palmar side

LI-4: *On the back of the hand, midway between the thumb*
and index finger, approximately 1 inch above the
web

Sp-10: *When the knee is flexed, 3 finger-breadths above*
the top edge of the patella, on the inside of the thigh;
feel for pain or tenderness at the spot

UB-40: *In the middle of the crease on the back of the knee,*
in the soft spot between tendons

TREATMENT FOR ACNE

Western Medicine Treatment

Conventional treatment for acne may include:

- Topical medications, such as retinoids, antibiotics, benzoyl peroxide, or salicylic acid
- Oral medications, such as antibiotics, Accutane® (isotretinoin), or (for women) birth control pills
- Chemical peels, dermabrasion, or laser treatment to help improve appearance of acne scars

Patients should discuss their treatment plan with their dermatologist.

Complementary and Alternative Treatment

Complementary therapies for acne may include:

- Nutritional therapy, including supplements with zinc, l-carnitine, or Vitamin A
- Topical ointments, such as with niacinamide, tea tree oil, witch hazel, azelaic acid
- Herbal remedies, such as guggul (an oral remedy)
- Ayurvedic medicine, which may involve a combination of special oral and topical treatments
- Homeopathic remedies, such as belladonna, calendula, hepar sulphur, kali bromatu, or silicea

Some of these treatments could have side effects. It is important for patients to be treated by a qualified health care professional.

NAET® Treatment

Different types of acne vary depending on the location, appearance, and contributing factors. When a patient suffers from an eruption of acne, the NAET® Specialist will look for the location corresponding with a meridian, then look at the appearance or shape of the acne. Then the NAET® Specialist will determine the exact allergen that lead to the acne manifestation using NAET® testing procedures. When a patient is treated with NAET® for the that allergen, the body will immediately produce the necessary chemical messengers and secretions (remedies) to open up the particular blockage in the particular energy pathway and reabsorb the accumulated lymph, cellulites, blood, pus, bacteria, etc. into the circulation, then eliminate them via urine or sweat.

NAET® treatment for acne involves desensitization for NAET® Basics and Classics as needed, then treating for the causative agent(s). Allergens commonly associated with acne include:

- Ingestants: Sugar, spices, deep fried foods, fried sweet foods (e.g., donuts) food additives, food colorings, animal fats, vegetable fats, grains
- Contactants: Feathers, cleansing agents, cosmetics, water, fabrics, hormones, stomach acids, digestive enzymes
- Infectants: Bacteria, fungus, parasites, yeast, *Candida*, contamination of the skin by infected agents
- Psychogenic causes: Emotional blockages

In addition:

- Poor digestion, poor elimination, and not drinking enough water can also contribute to acne.

- While going through the NAET® treatment program, patients may need some good supportive care (such as those described in Western and complementary approaches, above) to keep symptoms under control.
- Because NAET® treatments help eliminate accumulated lymph, cellulites, blood, pus, bacteria, etc. through the urine, patients should collect a sample of early morning urine and self-balance using the general balancing points (Figure 4-2) for the urine sample once daily.
- Patients should collect a sample of daily foods and self-balance using the general balancing points (Figure 4-2) every four hours until symptoms subside.
- Patients may also use acupressure self-help as described earlier in this chapter; the points specific to acne are shown in Figure 4-6.

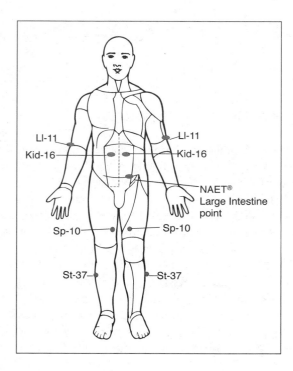

Figure 4-6.
Acupressure points
for ACNE.

Point locations:
Kid-16: *Half an inch to the side of the belly button*
NAET® LI point: *Three inches below and 4 inches to the left of center of the the belly button*
LI-11: *When the elbow is flexed, it is at the outside end of the elbow crease*
Sp-10: *When the knee is flexed, 3 finger-breadths above the top edge of the patella, on the inside of the thigh; feel for pain or tenderness at the spot*
St-37: *Six inches below the outside edge of the patella, on the line connecting the middle of the patella and the lateral malleolus (which is at the outside bony bump at the bottom end of the long bone in the lower leg)*

TREATMENT FOR PSORIASIS

Western Medicine Treatment

Psoriasis is a lifelong condition. Currently conventional treatment does not offer a cure, but various treatments can help to control symptoms. Many of the most effective agents used to treat severe psoriasis carry an increased risk of significant disease (e.g., skin cancer, lymphoma, and liver disease). However, most cases of psoriasis do not require that level of treatment. Most patients experience minor localized patches, particularly on the elbows and knees, which can be treated with topical medication. Patients often experience cycles of flare-up and remission throughout their lives, so controlling the signs and symptoms typically requires lifelong therapy. The patient's response to treatment will depend on many factors: location, extent and severity, age, gender, immune system status at the time of treatment, quality of life, and risks associated with the treatment.

Conventional treatment for psoriasis may include:

- Prescription topical medication, such as corticosteroids, salicylic acid, retinols, or calcipotriene
- Prescription oral medication, such as methotrexate, cyclosporine, soriatane, or biologics (made from human and animal proteins)
- Over-the-counter remedies, such as ibuprofen, petroleum jelly, coal tar ointments and shampoos, or capsaicin cream
- Phototherapy (ultraviolet radiation)

Patients should discuss their treatment plan with their dermatologist.

Complementary and Alternative Treatment

Complementary therapies for psoriasis may include:

- Nutritional therapy, such as eliminating alcohol, simple sugars, inflammatory fats (meat, dairy)
- Supplements, such as fish oil, Vitamin E, folate, zinc, selenium, grape seed extract, shark cartilage
- Herbal remedies, including supplements such as milk thistle, yellowdock, red clover, burdock, coleus forskohlii, evening primrose oil, or oregano oil; and herbal topical applications, such as aloe vera, apple cider vinegar, capsaicin cream, evening primrose oil, oats or oatmeal baths, tea tree oil, Oregon grape
- Homeopathic remedies, such as apis mellifica, calendula, rhus toxicodendron, sulphur
- Acupuncture treatments
- Chiropractic treatments
- Lifestyle changes, such as exercise, drinking plenty of water, or exposure to sunlight (wearing non-allergic sunscreen with an SPF of 15 or higher to avoid sunburn)
- Mind-body medicine for stress reduction

Some of these treatments could have side effects. It is important for patients to be treated by a qualified health care professional.

NAET® Treatment

NAET® treatment for psoriasis involves strengthening the immune system (treating with NAET® for Basic and Classic allergens), and avoiding and/or treating with NAET® for allergens commonly associated with psoriasis:

- Ingestants: milk and milk products (cottage cheese, yogurt, butter are major ones), spices (cinnamon, ginger, garlic), lemon, lime, orange, fermented foods
- Inhalants: chemicals
- Contactants: detergents, chemicals, fabric softeners, water, other household chemicals

In addition:

- Any allergen that makes the liver meridian weak is also associated with psoriasis.
- During NAET® treatments, patients should collect a sample of early morning urine and self-balance using the general balancing points (Figure 4-2) for the urine sample once a day.
- While going through the NAET® treatments, patients may need some good supportive care (such as those described in Western and complementary approaches, above) to keep symptoms under control.
- Patients should collect a sample of daily foods and self-balance using the general balancing points (Figure 4-2) every four hours until symptoms subside.
- Patients may also use acupressure self-help as described earlier in this chapter; the points specific to psoriasis are shown in Figure 4-7.

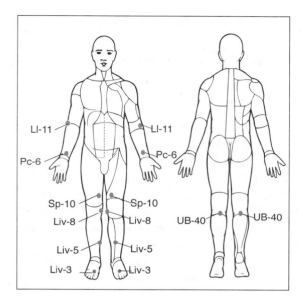

Figure 4-7.
Acupressure points
for PSORIASIS.

Point locations:

LI-11: When the elbow is flexed, it is at the outside end of the elbow crease

Pc-6: Three finger breadths above the wrist crease on the palmar side

Sp-10: When the knee is flexed, 3 finger-breadths above the top edge of the patella, on the inside of the thigh; feel for pain or tenderness at the spot

Liv-8: On the inside of the knee joint, behind the top edge of the tibia (which is the large long bone in the bottom part of the leg)

Liv-5: On the inside of the tibia (long bone in the bottom of the leg), 5.25 inches above the tip of the medial malleolus (which is the bony bump at the bottom end of the tibia)

Liv-3: On the top of the foot, in the soft spot between the end of the long bones of the 1st and 2nd toes

UB-40: In the middle of the crease on the back of the knee, in the soft spot between tendons

TREATMENT FOR CANDIDIASIS

———— ⟡ ————

Western Medicine Treatment

It is important to consider that *Candida* species are frequently part of the human body's normal oral and intestinal flora. Candidiasis is occasionally misdiagnosed by medical personnel as bacterial in nature, and treated with antibiotics against bacteria. This can lead to eliminating the yeast's natural competitors for resources, and increase the severity of the condition. But in clinical settings, candidiasis is commonly treated with antimycotics (antifungal drugs).

Just as there are different types of candidiasis, there are somewhat different ways to treat the disease.

- Oral candidiasis ("thrush") is commonly treated with a medicated (antifungal) liquid that is swished around the mouth and swallowed, or a lozenge that is sucked, dissolved in the mouth, and swallowed.
- Vaginal candidiasis ("yeast infection"), after confirmed by cultures, pH level check, and microscopic examination of vaginal secretions to rule out other possible infections, can be treated with medicated vaginal cream/suppositories or oral preparations, under the direction of the treating gynecologist; note that oral preparations should be avoided during pregnancy.
- Esophageal candidiasis is considered more severe and difficult to treat than oral thrush or vaginal yeast infections; patients should check with their doctor for treatment options with pharmaceutical support.

- Cutaneous candidiasis may be treated with topical anti-fungal medication. Oral antifungal, steroid, or antibiotic medication may be needed for *Candida*-associated folliculitis or nail infection.

Treating candidiasis solely with medication may not give desired results, and other underlying causes require consideration. Patients should discuss their treatment plan with their doctor.

Complementary and Alternative Treatment

Complementary therapies for candidiasis may include:

- Topical herbal remedies, such as gentian violet for oral candidiasis
- Direct application of yogurt (which contains lactobacillus), acidophilus salves, tea tree oil, lavender essential oil, calendula salve, or a mixture of honey, olive oil, and beeswax
- Nutritional therapy, such as eating a diet consisting primarily of green, fresh, raw vegetables, garlic (which yield allicin, an antifungal agent), nuts (essential fatty acids), whole grains (B vitamins), oregano, cinnamon, sage, and cloves (antifungal spices); no alcohol, no simple sugars, no yeast, and very limited amounts of refined foods and simple carbohydrates (even fruit juice)
- Supplements such as acidophilus and other probiotics, Vitamins C and B-complex, essential fatty acids, calcium, magnesium, caprylic acid, zinc, garlic
- Herbal remedies, such as Pau d'arco tea, Echinacea, goldenseal, fireweed
- Homeopathic remedies, such as borax, belladonna, chamomilla, arsenicum, graphites, or kreosotum
- Acupuncture treatment

Some of these treatments could have side effects. It is important for patients to be treated by a qualified health care professional.

NAET® Treatment

NAET® treatment for candidiasis involves strengthening the immune system (treating with NAET® for Basic and Classic allergens), and avoiding and/or treating with NAET® for allergens commonly associated with candidiasis:

- Ingestants: rice, wheat, corn, grains, sugar and sugar products, refined starches, coffee, chocolate, spices, deep fried foods, acidic foods, fruits, moldy food, salt, vegetables, nuts, processed foods, food colorings, food additives, food preservatives, vitamins, herbal supplements, hormone supplements, other drugs
- Contactants: wool, cotton, silk, polyester, acrylic, acetate, or other fabrics, silica, ocean water, rainwater, sanitary napkins, tampons, cotton crotches of underwear, pantyhose, toilet paper, body soap, detergent, skin creams, saliva, semen, vaginal mucus, other body secretions, bed linen, plastic bath toys and accessories, and pets

In addition:

- While going through the NAET® treatments, patients may need some good supportive care (such as those described in Western and complementary approaches, above) to keep symptoms under control.
- During NAET® treatments, patients should collect a sample of early morning urine and self-balance using the general balancing points (Figure 4-2) for the urine sample once a day.
- Patients should collect a sample of daily foods and self-balance using the general balancing points (Figure 4-2) every four hours until symptoms subside.

- Patients may also use acupressure self-help as described earlier in this chapter; the points specific to candidiasis are shown in Figure 4-8.

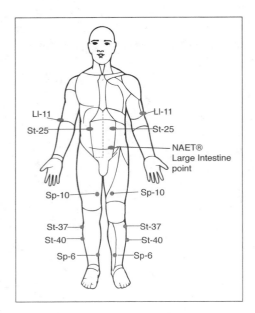

Figure 4-8.
Acupressure points for
CANDIDIASIS.

Point locations:

St-25: Three inches to the side of the center of the belly button

NAET® LI point: Three inches below and 4" to the left of the center of the belly button

LI-11: When the elbow is flexed, it is at the outside end of the elbow crease

Sp-10: When the knee is flexed, 3 finger-breadths above the top edge of the patella, on the inside of the thigh; feel for pain or tenderness at the spot

St-37: Six inches below the outside edge of the patella, on the line connecting the middle of the patella and the lateral malleolus (which is at the outside bony bump at the bottom end of the long bone in the lower leg)

St-40: Six inches above the lateral malleolus, and 2 finger-breadths to the side of front edge of the tibia (the long bone in the front part of the lower leg)

Sp-6: On the inside of the lower leg, 4 finger-breadths directly above the tip of the medial malleolus (which is the inside bony bump at the bottom end of the long bone in the lower leg)

TREATMENT FOR ATHLETE'S FOOT

Western Medicine Treatment

The tinea infections that cause athlete's foot may disappear spontaneously, or they can persist for years. Conventional treatment for athlete's foot may include:

- Topical preparation
- Multiple daily cleansing of the area
- Medicinal powder

However, these infections are particularly difficult to eliminate, even with attentive treatment and wearing light cotton socks to avoid further infection from dyes in the material. Best results usually are obtained with early treatment before the infection is firmly established. Antifungal or antibiotic medication (if the infection is actually bacterial, but looks like athlete's foot) may be prescribed. Patients should discuss the treatment plan with their doctor.

Complementary and Alternative Treatment

Complementary therapies for athlete's foot may include:

- Lifestyle changes, such as keeping the feet dry, changing socks frequently, wearing sandals or open footwear to expose skin to sunlight
- Topical application of tea tree oil or crushed raw garlic

NAET® Treatment

NAET® treatment for athlete's foot involves strengthening the immune system by desensitization for NAET® Basics and Classics. If it is a real case of athlete's foot (tinea pedis), it will clear with NAET® treatment for dermatophytes after completion of the Basics. Allergic reactions — such as from socks made of cotton, Orlon®, wool, or nylon — can mimic athlete's foot; in such cases, patients should eliminate the allergy with NAET® treatment for these fabrics so that athlete's foot-like symptoms can be reduced or cleared permanently. Other NAET® treatments that desensitize to other allergens commonly associated with athlete's foot include:

- Ingestants: baking soda, baking powder, corn starch, grains, sweets
- Contactants: sweat, MBT and mercaptothiazole (chemicals used in the socks by the industry while making socks to reduce odor), detergents
- Infectants: bacteria, parasites
- Molds and fungi

In addition:

- While going through the NAET® treatments, patients may need some good supportive care (such as those described in Western and complementary approaches, above) to keep symptoms under control.
- During NAET® treatments, patients should collect a sample of early morning urine and self-balance using the general balancing points (Figure 4-2) for the urine sample once a day.
- Patients should collect a sample of daily foods and self-balance using the general balancing points (Figure 4-2) every four hours until symptoms subside.
- Patients may also use acupressure self-help as described earlier in this chapter; the points specific to Athlete's Foot are shown in Figure 4-9.

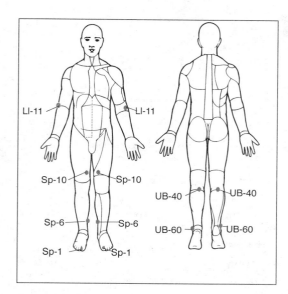

Figure 4-9.
Acupressure points for
ATHLETE'S FOOT.

Point locations:

LI-11:   When the elbow is flexed, it is at the outside end of
            the elbow crease

Sp-10:   When the knee is flexed, 3 finger-breadths above
            the top edge of the patella, on the inside of the
            thigh; feel for pain or tenderness at the spot

UB-40:   In the middle of the crease on the back of the knee,
            in the soft spot between tendons

Sp-6:   On the inside of the lower leg, 4 finger-breadths
            directly above the tip of the medial malleolus (which
            is the inside bony bump at the bottom end of the
            long bone in the lower leg)

UB-60:   In the soft spot below the lateral malleolus (which is
            at the outside bony bump at the bottom end of the
            long bone in the lower leg)

Sp-1:   On the medial side, 0.1" toward the heel from the
            corner of the toenail

TREATMENT FOR BALDNESS AND HAIR LOSS

Western Medicine Treatment

Conventional treatment for baldness or hair loss may include:

- Oral medications: finasteride (marketed for hair loss as Propecia®) and minoxidil, which are the only two treatments approved by the United States F.D.A. (Food and Drug Administration) for androgenetic alopecia, otherwise known as male or female pattern hair loss
- Symptomatic treatment might include corticosteroid medication

Treating doctors may also try to find the root cause, and eliminate the cause if treatable. In these cases, treatment may include:

- Antifungal medication
- Hormone supplementation
- Thyroid balancing medication

In some cases, surgical procedures such as hair transplants, scalp reduction or grafts may be an option. Patients should discuss their treatment plan with their doctor.

Complementary and Alternative Treatment

Complementary therapies for baldness or hair loss may include:

- Nutritional therapy, such as eating more fresh vegetables, whole grains, essential fatty acids, and non-animal protein; eating less of pro-inflammatory foods (e.g., saturated fats, dairy products)
- Supplements such as biotin, zinc, magnesium, Vitamins B6 and E, essential fatty acids such as Gamma-linolenic acid (GLA)
- Herbal remedies such as saw palmetto, beta-sitosterol, chase tree, Echinacea, astragalus, Siberian ginseng, or tea made from ginkgo, rosemary, prickly ash bark, black cohosh, yarrow, and horsetail; polygonum multiflorum (Shou Wu Pian) is a Chinese herb that is very effective in male pattern baldness, however one side effect is growing a beard, so it is not advised for females
- Mind-body medicine for stress reduction
- Massage to increase blood flow to the scalp

Some of these treatments could have other side effects. It is important for patients to be treated by a qualified health care professional.

NAET® Treatment

NAET® treatments may help reduce or slow the process of male pattern baldness if the underlying reason can be detected and treated. In addition to strengthening the immune system by desensitization for NAET® Basics and Classics, NAET® treatment for baldness or hair loss involves avoiding and/or treating with NAET® for allergens commonly associated with baldness or hair loss:

- Ingestants: nutrients
- Contactants: hormones, DNA and combinations, drinking water, water from the shower, bath towels, shampoo, hair conditioner, fabrics, hats, anything that contacts the head, and fallen hair
- Psychogenic causes: emotional stressors

In addition:

- NAET® emotional treatments can assist the individual to reduce the effects of emotional traumas and embarrassments associated with hair loss.
- While going through the NAET® treatments, patients may need some good supportive care (such as those described in Western and complementary approaches, above) to keep symptoms under control.
- Patients should collect a sample of daily foods and self-balance using the general balancing points (Figure 4-2) every four hours until symptoms subside.
- Patients may also use acupressure self-help as described earlier in this chapter; the points specific to baldness or hair loss are shown in Figures 4-10 through 4-12.

There is no one treatment or therapy made for everyone. Patients need to investigate all treatment options, and work with a qualified health professional to select the appropriate treatment plan for their condition.

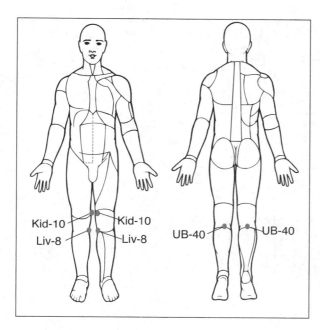

Figure 4-10.
Acupressure
points for
*BALDNESS
IN MEN.*

Point locations:

Kid-10: When the knee is flexed, the point is on the medial side of the knee joint, between the tendons of the hamstring muscles

Liv-8: On the inside of the knee joint, behind the top edge of the tibia (which is the large long bone in the bottom part of the leg)

UB-40: In the middle of the crease on the back of the knee, in the soft spot between tendons

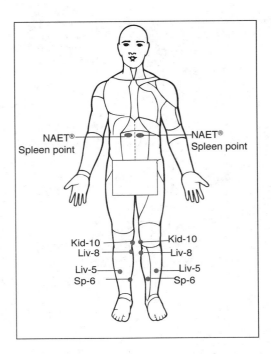

Figure 4-11.
Acupressure points for
BALDNESS IN WOMEN.

Point locations:

NAET® Sp point: On the abdomen, 3.75 inches above and 2 inches to the side of the belly button, on the lower border of the rib cage

Kid-10: When the knee is flexed, the point is on the medial side of the knee joint, between the tendons of the hamstring muscles

Liv-8: On the inside of the knee joint, behind the top edge of the tibia (which is the large long bone in the bottom part of the leg)

Liv-5: On the inside of the tibia, 5.25 inches above the tip of the medial malleolus (which is the inside bony bump at the bottom end of the tibia)

Sp-6: On the inside of the lower leg, 4 finger-breadths directly above the tip of the medial malleolus

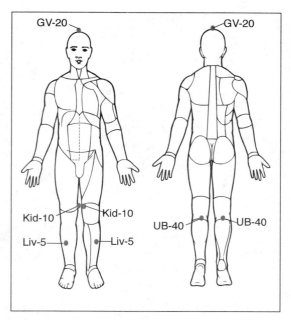

Figure 4-12.
Acupressure points
for *HAIR LOSS
AFTER
CHEMOTHERAPY.*

Point locations:

GV-20: Center of the top of the head

Kid-10: When the knee is flexed, the point is on the medial side of the knee joint, between the tendons of the hamstring muscles

UB-40: In the middle of the crease on the back of the knee, in the soft spot between tendons

Liv-5: On the inside of the tibia (long bone in the bottom of the leg), 5.25 inches above the tip of the medial malleolus (which is the inside bony bump at the bottom end of the long bone in the lower leg)

CHAPTER 5

A COLLECTION OF NAET® SUCCESS STORIES

Freedom from Allergies!

ECZEMA

Freedom From Eczema: Pam's Journey

I have had eczema since I was two days old. My mother died in childbirth and so I was given cow milk, however I was very allergic to lactose and the milk protein called casein.

Over the years, I have gone to doctors all over the country. I would itch so badly I would have to change my clothes several times daily because of the blood stains. I tried using black tar ointments, which would also stain my skin and clothes, as well as Benadryl™ and parabenzamine, which made me groggy.

Once when I was six years old I went into a public swimming pool and all the mothers took their children out of the pool. I felt like a leper. I got out of the pool and they went back in. I tried again; the same thing happened.

I did allergy testing and received shots for over 30 years, with many different doctors, and nothing helped. When cortisone be-

came available, it was a miracle! My skin cleared completely and I felt wonderful, but soon I was to gain over 40 pounds, got moon faced, a hump on my back, and who knows what it did to my insides. That was in the 1950s. I got the cortisone pills under control but still was dependent on cortisone ointment every day, supplemented with shots or pills when I just couldn't stand it.

I have gone to environmental health clinics and stayed in a porcelain trailer for months. The restrictions on my life were horrible. It was an artificial, unreal world. And it didn't work either. When I got off the plane, I had to go get a cortisone shot. I gave myself 21 shots a day and after a month gave that up because I got worse.

I tried elimination and rotation diets which are difficult and make you feel so restricted, as you watch every one else eat all those wonderful foods. At a dark restaurant, I accidentally put a baby tomato in my mouth. Even though I took it out I got just a squirt, and it immediately gave me an extreme reaction.

Finally a doctor in New Mexico told me to go see Dr. Devi Nambudripad. Here she was only a half hour from my home! When I came to her my skin was broken out from head to toe. The air hurt my skin so I kept covered up as much as possible. My skin was so inflamed, dry and parched; my face felt like the Sahara Desert. It hurt to smile. I would get what I call an internal sunburn. I would be red and hot, especially my face, and then it would be dry and flaky and peel just like from a sunburn. That's how I felt externally but internally it was lousy too. I felt completely exhausted from the allergy attacks and just plain icky and achy inside.

The first thing Dr. Devi had to do was treat me for every type of clothing because I was allergic to every fabric. I had always known I couldn't get near silk or wool but didn't realize I was even allergic to unbleached cotton. When I was five years old I had the measles and they put silk pajamas on me. I nearly died. It was my father's wedding night, and they spent the night at the hospital with me.

I used to get hypoglycemic reactions, especially, if I went without eating for a while. When Dr. Devi treated me for sugar, my body began releasing Candida into the skin. I had severe outbreak of eczema and itching. I also began feeling dizzy. Dr. Devi treated me for sugar, Candida albicans, Candida mix, yeast mix, alcohol and my own blood, first each of them alone, then different combinations of all these. I was treated for all the Basic allergens before she decided to treat for these combinations. That did it. Now I am 66 years old. My skin is almost completely clear. I eat everything. Occasionally I'll have a reaction. Dr. Devi is a gifted detective in finding out what is causing the reaction of the moment. She treats it, and the relief is incredible and instant. There are even times when I can figure out what is causing the problem and I can treat it myself by massaging my acupressure points as Dr. Devi has taught all of us (her patients), and it works to my amazement.

I don't feel restricted and I'm not taking medication and NO CORTISONE! I'm feeling great most of the time. I cannot thank Dr. Devi enough for developing this technique and above all sharing with all of us, so that we too can have a life in this world (66 years I suffered ...but because of Dr. Devi and her NAET®, I will not have to suffer from my allergies again).

Dr. Devi gives of her energy, time, and undivided attention. She is a caring, loving, compassionate doctor and indeed a great healer. Thank you God, for leading me to Dr. Devi and through her giving me Freedom to Live Again!

Pam Burns
Los Angeles, California, U.S.A.

Allergy and Eczema in Nils, Four Years Old

Since birth, Nils was bothered by several allergies. First cow milk allergy was seen and later several other allergies came along. It was a little drama for this little boy. After many years using hormones creams, in June 2006 we reached the stage where we had to find another solution. In June 2006 Nils' hands were completely open and hurt by the eczema. He had terrible pain and itching. The hormone creams and antibiotics didn't help anymore. A friend brought our attention to NAET® therapy and finally we searched on the internet and found Linda. When I explained to Linda the problem, we were happy she could help us in a short time.

When we came in, Linda said to Nils: "Nils, I am going to make your hands better, so you won't have the itching anymore." (Comment from Linda: *I can't imagine that I've said this, but the mom remembers it like this.) I thought, you dare, but finally it was true. It has been going very well with his hands, and Nils can now tolerate the products that he was allergic to. Before we went to Linda, when Nils touched something with his hands, if it contained egg his hands began to itch terribly. Now we are so far along that he eats eggs. Linda has treated Nils for several allergies and it is SUPER. Nils needed hay fever tablets, eye drops, and nose spray for hay fever, but after being treated by Linda, we don't have to use these anymore. What a delight. We have a different child, who finally sleeps through the night and who doesn't wake up because of the itching. Nils is four years old now.*

Linda, thank you.
Sylvia

NAET® Specialist: Linda Menkhorst
the Netherlands

My Daughter's Bleeding Eczema!

Our daughter Misha, (one-and-a-half years old at that time) had eczema. She had to sleep with her pajamas stitched so she couldn't scratch herself. Otherwise we would find her with open wounds and blood on her skin in the morning from scratching.

The itching was troubling her a lot. We read about NAET® through the internet. Then we found Karin, our NAET® practitioner.

After Karin treated Misha for egg mix, calcium mix, and Vitamin B-complex mix, she stopped scratching herself. There are still more allergens that have to be treated, but she is feeling already so much better and her skin looks much better. We decided to take a break. Moreover I was going to have another child. But when the summer started, the heat began bothering her. Her eczema returned.

Almost eight months later we returned helplessly to Karin for further assistance to reduce Misha's eczema. Misha was desperate. She itched severely through day and night. She couldn't sleep at night.

Karin examined her and said that she was reacting to the heat of the summer. She immediately treated her again one more time, this time for the heat. Her eczema disappeared once again!

Kind regards,
The Parents of Misha

Comment from Karin: *I got a phone call from the parents the following week after that last treatment for the heat. They said, "Misha is happy again, and her eczema has completely disappeared. NAET® is a miracle treatment! We love you!"*

NAET® Specialist: Karin Terwey
Holland, the Netherlands

Jasmijn Can Eat Everything Now

When Jasmijn was six months old she caught the RS [respiratory syncytial] virus. From that moment on she became allergic. Suddenly she couldn't handle dairy. For a while she was good with hypoallergenic dairy, but after a few month she got eczema on her back, which she scratched until she bled. We put her on a strict diet after a Nature health practitioner told us that she was allergic for milk, egg white, pork meat, citrus fruits, and tomato.

In two weeks all of her eczema disappeared. She held on to this diet for two years. We hoped she would grow out of it but that didn't happen. In August 2003 I read a story in a Dutch magazine about a boy and NAET®.

This therapy helped him to eliminate his allergies. We decided to try this therapy for Jasmijn, and visited Karin Terwey in Almere.

She tested her all over again with muscle testing. I (her mother) was the surrogate for Jasmijn because she was too young for the muscle tests. Jasmijn was allergic to calcium, milk, egg white, sugar, and pork meat. Each item was treated one by one, and after each treatment she had to stay away from the treated item for 25 hours. She wasn't allowed to touch or eat it in the 25 hours.

After seven treatments Jasmijn could eat everything without getting eczema.

Now, six months later, she can still eat everything. She isn't allergic anymore and can enjoy ice cream for the first time in her life.

Thanks Karin.

NAET® Specialist: Karin Terwey
Holland, the Netherlands

My Eczema Was From an Allergy to Fabrics!

A girlfriend told me about Karin Terwey and NAET®, because she treated her son's allergies. I had allergies so I visited her too. My complaints were: extreme tiredness every day, eczema, dry skin, and cuts on my fingers. First Karin treated me for some Basic allergens like sugar and minerals. After the sugar treatment I felt myself soon in better health. Further she treated me for fabrics, fabric colors, formaldehyde, and chemicals. My hands are no longer dry, the cuts are gone, and I can work with soap or washing powders without wearing gloves.

I'm so glad that NAET® helped me.
Thanks Karin.

NAET® Specialist: Karin Terwey
Holland, the Netherlands

Her Eczema Was From Environmental Allergies!

Tanya was four months old when she began to have eczema that covered her body. Her skin would crack, bleed, and get infected. We noticed it would get worse and that the itching progressed when we were outside. Doctors gave us many creams to try and we got no results from them. We heard of NAET® from a friend and gave it a try. It was really amazing to see her get treated for environmental things such as sunlight, heat, grass, etc. Her skin slowly healed and only a small spot on her thumb bothers her sometimes versus her entire body.

From the parents of Tanya

NAET® Specialist: Robert Prince, M.D.
Charlotte, North Carolina, U.S.A.

Freedom From Eczema

We found NAET® as an answer to my second daughter's eczema. Within three early treatments, Lianna's eczema had gone from a bleeding rash covering most of her body to an occasional redness behind her knees. I had also been having treatments for lifelong allergies and we were both enjoying the freedom that comes with NAET®.

That was until her new pets arrived: a rabbit and guinea pig that she didn't put down for days. Lianna's discomfort began showing up as restless nights. I was also itching and couldn't sleep. On the third night after the animals arrived at our home, Lianna woke up at 10 p.m. crying, hot, and itching, with inflamed eyes and a runny nose. I undressed her and she was covered in the eczema rash.

We were having dinner with friends, one of whom happened to be qualified in NAET®. Lianna and I were both allergic to the new pets and she treated us then and there. We both slept well that night, Lianna's symptoms resolved, the rash receded over the next few days, and I stopped itching. Since then, the animals are kissed and cuddled every day without any problem.

This is just one of many NAET® treatments I can be thankful for. Thanks Devi and the NAET® practitioners who have helped us here in Melbourne.

Lisa Bodley
Victoria, Australia

My Son's Eczema

Our son, now 14 years old, has been a lifelong allergy sufferer with asthma, eczema, and rhinitis. Over the years we have tried almost every form of treatment we could find – conventional medicine as well as Naturopathic remedies. Nothing seemed to make any difference. We even moved our family and home from Kentucky to Portland, Oregon in the hope that coastal environs would help – it did but for a limited time, and then the symptoms started coming back.

Last December, quite by accident, we came across NAET® on the internet. Upon probing further, we found a testimonial from Dr. Lisa Camerino in the NAET® Australian website. More importantly, Dr. Camerino, it turned out, was in Portland. We contacted her and started NAET® treatments in January of this year. The results have been near miraculous. Our son started to feel better after the first treatment and has continued to improve with subsequent treatments. Dr. Camerino with her practice of NAET® has affected our son's quality of life in a way that we have never experienced before – his eczema has improved, his rhinitis symptoms (when they arise) clear very quickly, and he is a much more relaxed person – his true personality is coming out. We are ever so grateful to Dr. Camerino and the NAET® process for all that it has done for our family.

We wish you and the NAET® foundation all the best. Please keep up the good work – you are making a huge difference to people like us in a very quiet way. We truly appreciate all that NAET® has done for our family.

Thank you,
Dr. Ashok & Banani
Portland, Oregon, U.S.A.

NAET® Specialist: Lisa Camerino, M.D.

My Daughter Is Free From Her Eczema!

My daughter was suffering from eczema so badly that she had open sores from it. Her doctor kept giving her topical ointments (with steroids in them) that kept "burning" her skin. I took her to see Dr. Chernoff, who took pictures of the sores, and cleared her of the lesions in a few visits. My daughter has scars from those sores, but she doesn't suffer from them anymore. As for myself, I started with clearing the food allergies, which in itself made me feel better. Not long after that, though, I started having a pain in my pelvis area. I went to see my doctor several times about it. She couldn't find anything wrong and told me to get up during the night to urinate and that would relieve the pain. Well, it didn't relieve the pain and every time I stood up to walk, a pain went shooting through me. I decided to see Dr. Chernoff and she immediately found that I had a gallbladder infection. After she treated me for it, I felt so good, no pain, no trouble urinating. Another thing she has helped me with recently is phantom pain. Since my amputation two years ago, I've felt like my phantom foot was always in a vice grip, gnarled up and throbbing with needles. Dr. Chernoff treated me for emotions connected to losing my leg and the Strep A/Staph *bacteria combination. During the treatment of the bacteria, I could feel the energy in my phantom leg release and it was as if my leg was there. It was such an awesome feeling! I have been making good progress towards feeling better and NAET® has helped in this process.*

Wanda M.

NAET® Specialist: Marilyn Chernoff, N.D., Ph.D., M.Ed.
Albuquerque, New Mexico, U.S.A.

We Conquered Bad Health, Eczema, and Allergies

My son Nordin was born on November 2, 2003. During the last weeks of the pregnancy I felt it didn't go well with him. In the hospital it was well watched. Afterwards it appeared that he had to fight hard until he was born (after 42 weeks). He gave it up at the last moment. Fortunately there were enough doctors around who saved his life three times. He was completely exhausted and had a lot of pain. Then he had to take medicine that kept him asleep for three months (he only woke up to drink now and then). But he grew well. After four months he became more restless, and at six months it really went wrong. He had eczema and seemed to be ill all the time. He cried nearly day and night. He had visible pain and was frightened because he couldn't breathe sometimes.

The doctors said he had all kinds of allergies and a bad immune system. And this could last until he would be seven years old.

We went to an osteopath, who treated him weekly. He cried less but remained ill.

When Nordin was one year old, and very weak, we visited Yolande van Rosmalen in Alkmaar, the Netherlands, who is a kinesiologist. Testing him she found many allergies.

Yolande treated me and that was very convenient for Nordin. We felt we were safe here. Yolande treated him every week and I saw him regaining his health. His skin was much better that summer, he didn't cry that much, and he ate and slept much better.

In autumn we stopped the treatments. In January he had pneumonia and went to the hospital. It was the first time he had a fever; now his immune system was working like it was the first time in his life. His lungs are much better now. I was convinced his immune system was working better than ever before.

*Last winter he only had a few colds. He has no allergies any-
more, and his skin is fine. He is developing very well now even
though the start of his life was a disaster. Even his doctor, who isn't
fond of alternative medicine, said he was doing very well.*

*Thanks to NAET®, we conquered bad health, eczema, and
allergies.*

Carla, a grateful mom

NAET® Specialist: Yolande van Rosmalen
Alkmaar, the Netherlands

A Childhood Event Caused Her Eczema!

*Mary Anne came to our office feeling like we were her last
hope. She had been to several doctors, including a dermatologist
and an alternative medicine practitioner. She wore only long sleeve
shirts and long pants because she was embarrassed about her skin
problems. Her skin was so red and inflamed that she felt like everyone avoided touching her. She had been diagnosed with eczema.
Mary Anne had read "Say Good-bye to Illness" and was hoping
that we would be able to help her. As Mary Anne went through her
initial Basic allergens treatments her skin started improving. The
redness started going away and her energy level starting improving. She continued with many treatments. Her treatment for amino
acids, and a chocolate allergy with an emotional component, were
very significant. Treating that emotional allergy turned out to give
the most profound shift in her symptoms. (When she was 10 years
old, her mother had asked her to watch her little sister. When she
was not looking, her four-year-old sister fell against the hot stove
and burned her one arm and the side of her face. Mary Anne felt
so guilty that she had let down her mother and her little sister got
hurt.) After we cleared the emotional allergy, 90% of her eczema*

went away. Her emotional allergy was causing physical symptoms on her skin.

NAET® Specialist: Cathy Goldstein Determan
Jacksonville Beach, Florida, U.S.A.

Whole Body Eczema in a 10-Year-Old Boy

In December of 2006 I began treating a 10-year-old boy who was covered in eczema. He had been to multiple traditional medical doctors as well as multiple holistic practitioners. He received moderate improvements with homeopathic treatment but it was not lasting. When he arrived in my office his arms, face, hands, and behind his knees were all extremely flared and raw from scratching. On testing, he was extremely weak on sugar, dairy, wheat, and food colorings treatments were done for each of these and sometimes multiple treatments were needed on each item. We then treated for specific foods that he enjoyed eating. After about 12 treatments, his mother stopped making appointments. Two months later I ran into his father who told me that the reason they stopped the treatments was because his son was completely cleared of his eczema. He looked like a different person and he was totally thrilled. His father tells everyone in the neighborhood that I am an angel! And he has referred many patients to me.

NAET® Specialist: Lisa Vecchi, N.D.
Oakville, Ontario, Canada

Eczema and Asthma

As a baby I developed eczema on my back and throughout my childhood had outbreaks behind my knees and in my elbows. At the age of five, I also developed asthma. These diseases were

*not very common at that time and my attacks were somewhat of a
novelty at school.*

*It was not until I was well into my teens that I developed hay
fever, and my asthma attacks began to last longer, and I also developed a form of weeping eczema. After a period in hospital with
a bad attack of asthma, I was prescribed Becotide® (a preventor)
and Ventolin® (a reliever) inhalers, which I have used ever since.
Approximately eight years ago my eczema began to get much
worse and eventually my dermatologist said that my immune system had completely broken down. At this stage I suffered from recurring abscesses in my teeth, which would not heal despite large
doses of antibiotics. It was then that my own doctor (a general
practitioner) and I felt that conventional medicine had no more
to offer me, and recommended me to a homeopath. Unfortunately,
under this regimen one has to get worse before one can get better
and, after discarding all medication except my inhalers, I developed eczema all over my body with the exception of my feet. For
the first three months I do not believe that I slept at all.*

*However after approximately two years I began to see great
improvement, but then suffered a massive asthma attack, which
put me into hospital for a second time. I believe that this attack
was due to a combination of unseasonably hot weather and the
flowering of the rapeseed crop. However, my homeopath was con-
cerned enough to consider that it was no longer safe to treat me.*

*I have since tried every other alternative you can think of with the
exception of herbal remedies, and all have played their part in making some improvement. However, 18 months ago, after yet another
deterioration in my condition, I was searching the internet and came
across NAET®. It was fortunate for me that two people had just begun
to practice in England, and I started my treatments in a weekly basis
in September 2000. It is now November 2001, and after approximately 60 treatments, I only have a small amount of eczema on my face
and hands, which is gradually reducing with every treatment. I have*

also never felt better in my life. For the last seven months, I have used my Becotide® inhaler for only one week (compared to having used it twice daily for 23 years); and, I have barely used my Ventolin® at all, even through the rapeseed season, which was when I always suffered the most.

I cannot recommend this treatment highly enough. It gets to the cause of the allergy (extremely important when it comes to environmental allergens), does not merely mask the symptoms, and is the only treatment I have tried where I have been encouraged to continue use of relieving medication while having treatment. The best thing is of course, after the first 25 hours, you don't have to avoid the allergen anymore!

NAET® Specialist: Julie Holland, B.S.Y.A. (Kin.)(Acu.)(A.P.)
Leicester, Liecs, England
European practitioner: Pamella Bretell
Cambridge, England

Eczema and Dry Skin

A nine-year-old girl had eczema with severe dry skin that would crack and bleed. It would bleed more than once per week. She had severe allergy to citrus. Exposure would cause increased rash and illness for one to two weeks.

We treated her for milk and Vitamin C, and the next day she was eating citrus with NO reactions. Within two days her skin was like a new baby's skin. Her eczema was gone within two days of the citrus treatment.

NAET® Specialist: David R. Pinkston, D.C.
St. George, Utah, U.S.A.

Melatonin Causing Eczema in My Two-Year-Old

My little two-year-old daughter started getting eczema on her legs. Her skin felt like fine sandpaper and was reddening on her thighs with a line of demarcation ending at her cloth diaper. As it worsened she actually had welted/raised areas on her thighs that were very red and inflamed. She also had very bad areas on the backs of her hands and on the inside of her wrists. She was always scratching. She was even biting the insides of her wrists when they were bad. She had scabby areas from scratching. As her skin worsened so did her mood. She would have trance-like crying spells where she would throw herself back on the floor and kick her feet screaming and crying. Nothing would bring her out of the crying except letting her cry for a bit. Tiny strange things would set her off, like my picking out the wrong outfit for her to wear or moving her plate closer to her while she was eating. If we tried to engage her to play with us, she would resist. She only wanted to play if it was her choice. Poor impulse control was associated with the crying spells, biting, hitting, and scratching when upset. Her threshold for frustration was so very low. She was very clingy when upset (of course). She wanted to be carried everywhere. She would say, 'Up, mama, up, mama' when she was upset. When she did cheer up, she was very happy. So it was all very Jekyll and Hyde. She was also very picky about eating. The food was always the wrong food, the wrong amount, and she would actually get so upset she would impulsively throw her fork or spoon, or even her glass of water to get it away from her. Then, she would cry for the food that she threw away from herself. Every meal was a nightmare. She was also having a very difficult time going to sleep. She would lie down and very patiently try to fall asleep. She would close her eyes and relax, but it would take hours for her to finally drift off. Once she fell asleep, though, she would sleep well. Her bowel movements were VERY smelly and full of undigested food. Finally, she had a huge long crying spell of 30 minutes or so. It was awful. She was so hysterical and nothing I did would calm her down.

Dr. Marilyn Chernoff determined that it was the hormone Melatonin that was giving my daughter so much trouble. She treated her that day. In the morning I looked at her skin and the eczema was still there, but the raised areas were completely flat and her skin was no longer red and she was scratching much less! That morning she ate breakfast without incident. She seemed calmer and happier and was playing with her sister without arguing. Her mood was much smoother all day, and even though she was a bit fussy, she had no crying spells at all. That night she fell asleep so easily and quickly even before the nighttime story was over. The next day her skin was smooth and much healed. She actually had soft skin in lots of places. The fine sandpaper feel was gone. There was no redness and the little scabs were gone and healed. She was only scratching occasionally. Her bowel movements were much improved and she was eating foods again without incident as well as sitting happily with us at the table without incident. At the end of this second day I noticed I felt like something was missing. Oh yes, it was my 25-pound child. She wasn't in my arms all day and they felt empty.

NAET® Specialist: Marilyn Chernoff, N.D., Ph.D., M.Ed.
Albuquerque, New Mexico, U.S.A.

Cow Milk and Eczema

As a small child, my patient had eczema behind her ears. When her mother stopped giving her cow milk, the eczema disappeared. At the age of 13 the eczema came back at the elbow, the back of her knees, and behind the ears. From age 13 to 19, the eczema developed all over her body, getting worse. Finally she had a blood test showing that she was allergic to egg, milk, nearly all kinds of meat and fish, shellfish, wheat, and some pollen from trees and plants. She started a diet and avoided all the items she was allergic to. Her skin got better, but the eczema never disappeared completely.

Three years ago the eczema was getting worse again, mainly on the hands and arms. When she came to me, we started with all of the Basic allergens and found many items she reacted to. We went through the pollen and fruit-mix. But the eczema was still there on her hands and arms. This patient is now a physical therapist, and therefore she often has contact with oil on the skin. After treating these items, the eczema on the hands and arms finally improved.

NAET® Specialist: Claudia Lanting-Lehn
Zandvoort, the Netherlands

Atopic Dermatitis

One of my patients brought her younger sister to my office. She had suffered from atopic dermatitis for about 17 years. As a chiropractor, I could have never accepted this type of patient prior to learning NAET®. Basic NAET® training provided me enough confidence to address her present condition. Other than the classroom training I received in NAET®, I did not have any first-hand experience in treating skin conditions. I decided to face the challenge. I did my best to treat her and eventually I got very successful results. Therefore I would like to report about this case study as an encouraging endeavour to beginning NAET® practitioners, to give them some confidence to accept the challenge. I took the Basic seminar in January 2005 for the first time. Three weeks later I began treating this challenging case.

Case: 27-year-old female office worker

Chief complaint: Atopic dermatitis

History: Onset during third grade. She went to her dermatologist and he prescribed ointment for her itching. Her symptom had occurred intermittently and gradually became worse. She changed her job at the age of 22. This new job put a severe stress on her especially because she was incompatible with her boss. This environment made her skin disorder worsen further. She began to use a steroid ointment with no result. She had been also prescribed an antidepressant and sleeping pills since the age of 23. She suffered from severe menstrual pain since then as well.

First consultation: Late January 2005. The patient's facial expression was very stiff probably due to stress from her job. Severe atopic dermatitis was seen at her neck, lower and upper extremities, hip, lower abdomen, and chest. It looked like cholesterol oxide dermatitis. Before starting treatment, I explained about the threat of corticosteroids and suggested her to consult with her dermatologist for the possibility to wean off from steroids gradually. She agreed with my opinion. I treated BBF on her first visit.

Findings: Atopic dermatitis in this case was prominent in the area of the left hip, left anterior thigh, left dorsal hand, and left knee especially two weeks after she quit the steroid ointment. This may be due to rebound phenomenon. (Photos are omitted due to lack of space.)

Treatment: We proceeded with NAET® treatments. As she quit the steroid ointment, the rebound phenomenon was at its peak around her fifth visit to my office. After Vitamin A mix was cleared, the symptom became stable. After hormones were cleared, her menstrual pain was greatly reduced. In early summer her itching became worse and I found that various dusts might be related to this change. After several dusts and fats were cleared, she became mentally stable and quit the antidepressant.

Her atopic dermatitis became much better during that summer even though during this season she had always suffered from severe symptoms such as eczema, rashes, blisters, and erosion. She changed her job, got a boyfriend, and then quit using sleeping pills. As of September 30th, her skin disorder was almost completely reduced.

Discussion: As a beginner of NAET®, I was hesitant to accept this complicated case. Once I decided to treat her, I followed NAET® instructions and protocols very precisely, often reading the class notes many times prior to seeing her. She had suffered for 17 years without getting any help from anywhere. I was taught in the class that NAET® was able to produce significant improvements in cases like this. If it happened to others it could happen in her case too. I decided to try my best to find out the answer. When she was weaned off from cortisone, I observed the rebound phenomenon. I had not seen that in a patient before. I also learned the significance of the doctor's conviction, a trusting relationship between doctor and patient, the true meaning of the healing process, and the interactive relationship of body and mind. NAET® is amazing! I would like to devote more time to learn all about NAET® so that I would be more skillful with NAET® to get the maximum results in as short a period of time as possible.

NAET® Specialist: Shigeki Nakai, L.B.S.
Hirakata City, Osaka, Japan

Allergic Dermatitis

This patient came to my office not for seeking relief of allergic dermatitis, but for her low back pain. During treatment of her symptom I recognized the rashes on her neck and left wrist. I tried to get her consent to do NAET® treatments to help her rashes by explaining about NAET®. She accepted my offer and then I began to treat her skin disorder using NAET®.

Case: 28-year-old female office worker

Chief complaint: Low back pain
Other symptoms: Rashes at the neck and left wrist

History: The rashes appeared at age of 23. She felt itching after she got warm by taking a hot bath or after sweating. Her neck reacted to clothes, pillows, soap, and shampoo, resulting in rashes. The wristband of her watch and/or the sleeves of her clothes made her feel itchy. The symptom flared up especially during sleep and she scratched her skin with resultant bleeding. Her dermatologist prescribed steroids, which worked for her one time but not another time. She gave up attempting to cure this disorder. The onset of the rashes seemed to correspond to a stressful period in her life after she began working for her parents' company during a family feud.

First consulting: The rashes on her neck appeared to be solid skin and looked slightly purple. Red rashes were accompanied by bullous edema at her left wrist. I treated BBF only at this time (February 16, 2005).

Treatment: The NAET® treatments are listed according to the order of treatments given. Her last treatment was on September 30, 2005.

The Order of Treatments Given

1. BBF
2. White rice
3. Egg mix
4. Egg mix
5. Egg mix
6. BBF
7. Egg yolk
8. Egg white
9. Vitamin C mix
10. BBF
11. Vitamin B-complex
12. Vitamin A mix
13. Yeast mix
14. Yeast mix
15. Hormones
16. Iron mix
17. Hormones
18. Hormones
19. Salt mix
20. Hormones
21. Salt mix
22. Salt mix
23. Dust
24. Home dust
25. Job dust
26. Environment dust
27. Animal fat
28. Animal fat
29. BBF
30. Vegetable fat

31. Tap water	42. Clothes
32. Beef	43. Eel
33. Beef	44. Mineral water
34. Vitamin E	45. Chocolate
35. Vitamin D	46. Shrimp
36. Amino acids	47. Shrimp
37. Citrus mix	48. Ragweed
38. Caffeine mix	49. Blood
39. BBF	50. Blood
40. Animal dander	51. Estrogen
41. Spice-2	

Items Treated and Response Observed

Item	Response
Egg mix	Skin color on the neck came back to normal
Calcium mix	Itching subsided at her neck and wrist
Egg mix & Ca mix	Itching was totally gone
Vitamin C mix	Itching at her neck appeared again
Vit.C w/E, B-complex	No change
Sugar mix	Itching at her neck subsided
Sugar w/E, Iron	No itching at her neck. Skin color improved
Vitamin A mix	No itching
Mineral mix	No itching
Mineral w/E, Salt	Slight bollous edema at the wrist
Salt mix again	Bollous edema subsided
Grain mix	Bollous edema and its itching subsided
Grain mix again	Termination of NAET® treatment

Result: Rashes at her neck and left wrist had subsided.

Discussion: Yeast mix, acid, base, and hormone, of the NAET® Basic allergens, still need to be treated. However this patient wanted to terminate the NAET® treatments due to personal rea-

sons. *Although I did not know the major culprit for this disorder, I followed the NAET® Basic allergen protocol faithfully with excellent results. Now I do realize why NAET® protocol stressed on the Basic allergen treatments before treating anything else. The Basic allergen group includes most essential nutrients needed for the body to grow properly, to supply adequate nutrients for growth and development, to eliminate toxins naturally, to repair the wear and tear that takes place almost everyday in the body and even to reduce allergic reactions from other substances. Now I believe in the significance of the NAET® Basic allergen samples.*

Tomoyuki Kono, B.C.Sc., L.B.S.
Itabashi-ku, Tokyo, Japan

Dermatitis From Vitamin C

D.G., a 50-year-old female, complained of a rash over her entire body. She stated that she was unable to get a good night's sleep due to her persistent itching. After receiving a treatment for Vitamin C her rash disappeared and she now enjoys a good sleep.

NAET® Specialist: Cheryl Cameron, R.N.P.
North Tetagouche, New Brunswick, Canada

More on Eczema...

A 19-month-old girl suffered from eczema and itching all over her body since she was six weeks old. After a blood test in a hospital, her mother knew that her daugther was allergic to milk, proteins, chicken, soya, peanut, dog and cat hair, pollen, and dust.

After the first NAET® treatment (BBF), using the mother as a surrogate, the itch disappeared!

Then I treated all the other items I found her allergic to. The eczema got better and her skin recovered.

*A **little girl** had a very dry and rough skin for about three years. Testing her for the first five NAET® Basic allergens, I found her allergic to egg mix, calcium mix, and milk mix. She needed to be treated for calcium three times, but then her skin recovered and got smooth.*

*A **12-year-old boy** had eczema at the back of his knees for about three years. After testing, I found him very allergic to latex and several kinds of rubber. When I finished three treatments for latex and rubber, he still tested weak on the emotional level with rubber. So I started searching for the emotional blockage. When he was a baby he had surgery in a hospital. The anaesthesia was done with a rubber chap covering his nose and mouth. After the emotional treatment for this incident, the itching rash disappeared.*

*An **18-month-old boy** presented with severe eczema all over his body with weeping, raw sores. He was always scratching his skin creating more problems. His mother knew he had severe food allergies to egg, corn, wheat, and other foods. She was making him abstain from these foods. He was on a very limited diet. Even though he was avoiding these foods his skin was very inflamed.*

The patient was treated for all of the NAET® Basic allergens, as well as soybean and tomato. His skin is completely smooth and beautiful now.

He had an emotional blockage to egg because it had made him feel so terrible in the past when he ate it. We treated several incidents before he was cleared for egg. Otherwise, he passed each treatment easily. His personality has really changed also. He used to be very fussy with lots of screaming and crying when he came to the office. Now he is so happy.

ACNE

—————————⟨⟨⟨⟨—————————

Freedom From Acne

A 26-year-old male came to me with the following complaints: he suffered from frequent outbreaks of huge painful, angry looking acne on his face or in different parts of the body at least once a week for years. There was no definite number of eruptions or specific area for them to appear. Sometimes he got them (may be one or two huge ones only) on his face just below the cheek bone, sometimes on his back (upper aspect of his scapula usually on either left or right side), below the neck, on the abdomen around the navel, in the inguinal region, and inside part of one thigh on either side about three inches below the groin area; these were the usual acne sites for him. Always he woke up with the acne, most often it happened on a Saturday morning. By the evening it might get as large as a grape with a red or white head and extremely painful. He used hot moist packs, antibacterial creams, and poultices. In a day or two it turned into pustules and eventually it would break and the pus would drain out giving some relief from his excruciating pain. The acne would heal by leaving a scar. He had accumulated several such scars on his face and body over the years. Eventually some of them faded away with the use of fade cream, etc. He has had several types of treatments for acne and repair of scars by various specialists around the world. He took various vitamins, minerals, antioxidants, and other supplements hoping to prevent further acne eruptions. But his acne continued to appear without any warning every now and then. He came in with a huge acne on his upper back on the right side. When I examined him through NAET® testing procedures, he was found to be very allergic to olives and garlic. He ate Italian food once a week, mainly on Friday night. Sometimes he ate pasta with garlic sauce, or other times he ate pizza with black olives. The night before his appointment with me he had eaten pasta with garlic sauce, one of his favorites. Garlic caused an energy imbalance (block) in his small intestine meridian resulting in skin eruptions under the cheek bones, below the neck, above the scapula, around the navel area. Olives caused an energy imbalance in the liver meridian resulting in the acne eruptions in the inguinal area or inside the thighs. His garlic sauce supper on the previous night and acne eruption on his upper back in the morning confirmed my NAET® diagnosis. Going through years of pain and agony, this young man wanted some proof or published studies before he could believe in the NAET® approach. He could not understand how his painful acne could get better without some kind of medication. I decided to put him through a simple experiment with his cooperation.

He had various allergies and health problems other than acne. He was started on NAET® treatments for Basic allergens. In the meantime, he was advised to eat pasta with garlic sauce for the following couple of weeks and was asked to record his symptoms. Both weeks the acne appeared on the left side below the cheek bone and above the left scapula. He was careful to eat a small quantity of pasta each time, so he got small acne lesions on both instances. Then he was advised to eat pizza with black olives on the following Friday. He was careful again and ate only a small piece of pizza and to his amazement, sure enough he got a small painful acne on his thigh. He was advised to eat a couple of pieces of pizza on the following week and was asked to bring a sample of the exact pizza on the next morning to the office for treatment. By this time he had completed Basic treatments and was ready to treat the pizza. The second time when he ate a couple of pieces, he developed a couple of huge grape-sized acne on his inside thighs and one in the groin, making regular walking difficult due to pain. He was treated for the pizza with black olives immediately and was left with acupuncture needles for an hour. Forty eight hours after the treatment, he reported to the office with a beaming smile on his face. He said he watched the acne very closely this time and he just rested in bed without any creams after he left my office. He said he wanted to understand the NAET® process and wanted to give NAET® a chance to do the job naturally. He continued to have severe pain for six hours but refused to take the usual analgesics or hot moist packs. Six hours after the NAET®, his pain gradually began to diminish and the size of the acne also reduced. Around 12 midnight when he woke up, he still felt the pain at the site of the acne. But when he woke up in the morning, he didn't feel any pain at all and when he looked at the acne, they were gone without leaving any sign on the skin. His body sucked the pimples in and normal skin appeared in their places. He was very thrilled with the result and he was sad that he had to wait until Monday evening before he could come to the office and share this exciting news with us. He was thoroughly convinced about the results of NAET®. He found a new way to overcome his health problems. He continued to treat for the next year and half for all allergens tested weak by Kinesiological methods (Neuromuscular Sensitivity Testing). He has not had another acne episode since then (for the past eight years now).

Acne From Vitamin A Deficiency

My daughter, Allison, had a goose-bump like rash on her arms and thighs for a few years. When reading in my nutrition course that this type of rash is caused by a Vitamin A deficiency, I boosted her for Vitamin A through NAET® and a few days later she came to me and said "I think I need another boost, my rash is almost all gone." I boosted her for Vitamin A again and the rash cleared up.

NAET® Specialist: Cheryl Cameron, R.N.P.
North Tetagouche, New Brunswick, Canada

The Chronic Acne on My Chin Is No More!

Remember the acne I had in New York this summer? It's all gone. I think the NAET® detoxing treatment is what did it! I detoxed glucose several times. The first time I was extremely fatigued for 25 hours, then a few days after, my right arm became VERY sore. I thought I was going to have to stop my NAET® practice for awhile, as that is the arm I use to perform NST. I thought I would have to go have a cortisone shot! I kept thinking in my head "I preach NAET® to everyone and tell them how wonderful it is, and here I am, suffering with a sore arm". I checked using QRT, and found that I had to do a second glucose detox. After the 25-hour period my arm was COMPLETELY pain free! I couldn't believe it, but was very glad to have experienced the discomfort to see how powerful the NAET® detoxification can be! I had to do a further glucose detox after that, and I cannot believe how the acne on my chin has cleared up!

My husband lost his mother about a month ago, and a few days after she left to go to a hospital for lung surgery, he developed a kidney stone. He was diagnosed at the hospital emergency room, and they gave him analgesics, an anti-inflammatory, and an antispasmodic, presuming that the stone would pass on its own. It didn't. He had three x-rays before he went to lithotripsy (several weeks later in which time he visited the family doctor and a urologist) to have it blasted. During this time I was detoxing him and doing NAET® treatments. When he went for the lithotripsy they gave him an x-ray to see where the stone was located (in case it had moved). They could not find it. The specialist thought he may have passed it, but my husband asked him if he would feel it being passed. He was assured that he would have felt it. They put in a dye and saw where the stone had moved along the urethra, then all signs of the stone disappeared, as did the stone. I had detoxed him for lead (he works at a lead smelter), caffeine, and several other things. Apparently the stone had dissolved!

Thanks for teaching us how to detox people with NAET®!

NAET® Specialist: Cheryl Cameron, R.N.P.
North Tetagouche, New Brunswick, Canada

My Rosacea Said Good-bye, Hopefully Forever!

I am a 26-year-old woman who has suffered with various allergies for the last nine years. Along with some food and pollen allergies, I suffered from acne rosacea. The rosacea would cause redness around my nose, which the doctor told me was caused by stress. I had tried several medicated creams, none of which worked very well. Upon hearing about NAET® from several people who had tried it with successful results, I thought 'why not?' My purpose was to eliminate my food and pollen allergies, however something very surprising happened. Not only are my allergies gone, so is my rosacea. Since my treatments, my nose has been cleared of redness and it has not returned as of yet. (I anticipate that it won't!)

Thanks to Cheryl and NAET®, my quality of life is much better than ever.

Thank-you Cheryl!
Eleanor Brown

NAET® Specialist: Cheryl Cameron, R.N.P.
North Tetagouche, New Brunswick, Canada

PSORIASIS

My Psoriasis Completely Disappeared After NAET®!

Since the NAET® treatments I received last December, the psoriasis that had been plaguing me for almost a year has almost completely disappeared. I have only a few itchy areas on my scalp and two small persistent areas of redness on my right cheek. This is down from total body involvement in December. I did and still do use other complimentary medical modalities such as: maintaining an alkaline diet, colonic irrigations, regular meditation, exercise, and massage. I must say however, that I experienced the most dramatic reduction in symptoms after NAET® treatments. I have continued to use only the products that I cleared with NAET® desensitization. The relief I have experienced is tremendous. Judging from other psoriasis sufferers I have met, my recovery is unusual in that I continue to improve with no flare-ups to date.

Sincerely,
Judy and Ken Nelson, Oregon, U.S.A.

Seven Years of Psoriasis

I suffered from psoriasis and joint pains for seven years. My skin completely cleared up after I was treated by Dr. Devi for calcium mix, cheese mix, chocolate, and vitamin F (fatty acids).

Theresa B.
Long Beach, California, U.S.A.

CANDIDIASIS

My Candidiasis, Fever Blisters, Cough, and More Are Gone After NAET®!

My body had become very systemically ill. I had a chronic cough that appeared untreatable. After every meal, everything I ate caused copious amounts of mucus and a 40-minute hacking, coughing, and blowing episode. I couldn't lose weight no matter how hard I tried. I got fever blisters repeatedly, and bronchial infections over and over. My regular medical doctor was baffled. I suspected allergies and had a blood allergy test run called Alcat (mentioned in the book Say Good-bye to Illness*), and I started doing research on different allergy treatments when I stumbled onto www.naet.com. I liked what I read, and I immediately bought the book. After reading the book I looked for a practitioner in my state. The closest one was one and a half hours away, but I made an appointment and it was the best thing I ever did. Karen Marshall is an extremely intuitive practitioner and NAET® works very well for me. I am really in tune to my body and what it needs, and I knew what I was allergic to but I didn't want to admit it. The Alcat test confirmed most of what I already knew, and then the muscle testing that Karen did during my first visit with her further confirmed the same findings. I told her I had done the Alcat test, but we didn't compare the results until the end, and they were almost identical with a few new ones added.*

Karen is great to work with. My body really takes to the treatments, so she is able to group treatments together and I often do two in the same day to save me the drive time. I have one treatment left and I feel amazing. She said she had never seen someone with as many allergies as I had. I was allergic to every sugar, every grain, Candida, *every mold, most trees, most dairy, and over 30 chemicals. I was even allergic to lemons and a few other foods. She went through the Basic allergens in order, and then we have been dealing with the environmental allergies. After I am finished we will check for any we missed the first time, but I can tell you I no longer cough at all, I only blow my nose once after I eat (I don't know if this will ever stop), and my body just feels well again. The best news is that weight is just falling off, and I still get to eat food I like though I do need to make better choices. Presently I am doing a yeast cleanse to get it out of my body now that I am cleared, and that is not a fun diet but I look forward to getting to eat some of my favorite foods again. I have promised to give up diet cola (any soft drink for that matter), processed flour, and sugars, but I can have other real sweeteners. I have found I have almost totally lost my sweet tooth. Also spelt bread is a good thing.*

An example of how it works: When I found out what I was allergic to, I stopped eating everything that was on my list while I waited the two weeks till I could get in for my first treatment. I did a colon cleanse and went through some of the negative symptoms that occur when you cleanse, and by doing that I have avoided most of the effects of the treatments. However during those two weeks, I really had a hankering for onion rings so when we went out to dinner I ordered some. It was the worst reaction I had ever had. Karen said it was because I had cleared my body but I was still allergic to the item. I almost had an asthma attack the mucus dump was so intense. I had an immediate five-pound gain that lasted for a week and I felt horrible.

After she cleared the grains and most of my other food (I was sure the ingredients of onion rings had been cleared), I decided to try it again and I had absolutely no reaction at all. I haven't had a mucus dump in over a month, and though I do feel the need to blow my nose after eating it, I only need to do so once.

She has taught me how to test my self with a test where you hold the item in front of you and close your eyes. If your body wants to weave forward, that is an okay item, and if it wants to weave backwards, stay away from the item. I have gotten so proficient at this test I can do it in about two seconds. Nothing comes in my house if I am allergic to it.

I know it sounds too good to be true, but believe me, it is true. I guess there are some people who are not testable, but I encourage people to go in with an open mind and find a practitioner who will work with you and make you well again. Above all, follow the rules of the treatment, and don't cheat. Anybody can do anything for 25 hours.

Sheila B.
Bloomington, Indiana, U.S.A.

NAET® Specialist: Karen S. Marshall, N.D., C.N.H.P., R.N.
Fishers, Indiana, U.S.A.

Candida albicans

I had Candida albicans, *a severe case of yeast in my blood, for over seven years. During that time I spent over $20,000 in out-of-pocket plus insurance expenses. Two of my doctors said that I would never get over it, even by staying on a rigid yeast-free diet, taking medications, injections, and intravenous feedings. Six months after I started seeing Dr. Devi Nambudripad for NAET® treatment, I could see the light at the end of the tunnel. Now I am beyond the end of the tunnel. Now I have been completely free of my* Candida *and yeast problem for the past 15 years.*

Charles Depoin
Laguna Beach, California, U.S.A.

VARIOUS SYMPTOMS
GONE AFTER NAET®

Itching on the Scalp Is Gone After NAET®!

NAET® treatments have made a huge difference in how I feel, and in what I can eat. I suffered from the oral allergy syndrome, and was unable to eat raw fruits, some nuts, soy, and sulfites. I am now able to enjoy all of the things I have been treated for, and just the other day ate a delicious plum and a pear. I am no longer afraid of having an allergic reaction when I eat out in restaurants. This peace of mind is priceless!

As I went through my treatments, I noticed many other benefits, beyond what I had initially gone to NAET® for. My persistently itchy scalp no longer wakes me up at night. I haven't had a panic attack in over a year, fear and anxiety are no longer dominating my life, and I am a much calmer, more energetic person. Much happier, too!

Debra is incredibly patient, and thorough. She is kind and understanding, and truly has her clients' best interests at heart. She is an ethical practitioner, and she continually updates her training and strives to give her clients the best treatments possible. I am fortunate to have found her, and have recommended her to many friends and family members.

My son has had a few NAET® treatments so far, and I have already noticed a big difference in his energy level and mood. He used to wake up very sluggish in the morning and have a hard time getting going. Now he is ready to go! His energy levels are much higher during the day, and he is on a more even-keel emotion-ally. When my daughter had her braces put on last year, I noticed that she went from being quite robust, to picking up every cold that came along. I took her to see Debra for NAET® testing, and sure enough, she was allergic to her braces. She will be treated for that allergy soon, and I am sure that this winter, her immune system will be much stronger and able to fight off colds. She has responded well to the other allergy treatments she has had so far. Her ragweed allergy cleared up after only one treatment!

Pam L.

NAET® Specialist: Debra Lowe, B.A., D.Ac.
Ottowa, Ontario, Canada

My Dry Skin

Thank you so much for treating me for oxytocin/pitocin. My skin was very dry. I hated even taking a shower because I knew I would itch afterward. My hands looked like an old relief map or something and I just couldn't moisturize them enough. Creams just wouldn't penetrate the surface to make them smooth. For a month I had small itching bumps in my hairline. I kept thinking they'd disappear, but then I got one in my eyebrow. When you treated me for oxytocin/pito-cin, all of this completely disappeared. My skin is smooth again! And my hands are MY hands again. I can style my hair without pain, and the itchy painful bumps are gone without a trace! Thank you so much. I am back to my happy, normal routine because of NAET®.

Annie

NAET® Specialist: Marilyn Chernoff, N.D., Ph.D., M.Ed.
Albuquerque, New Mexico, U.S.A.

Itchy, Inflammatory Rashes, and Hair Loss

I happened to read about NAET® and came here with a seri-ous skin condition called Lichen Planus. I had rashes all over my body and my both palms were affected with severe infection. When I came here and started NAET®, I also had itching which was un-bearable. The treatment helped me so much that my severe itching almost stopped, and my skin condition has improved a lot. After 31 treatments, I'm also seeing noticeable results such as improved nail growth, which is I'm sure is the result of calcium absorption. Also my hair loss has reduced, and in general I feel that my overall health has improved a lot after starting NAET®. I found NAET® at the right time and I'm very grateful to Sister Naina. All these were made possible with ever-smiling and encouraging support of Sister Naina. Thank you so much. Regards, Madhu Govindrajan

NAET® Specialist: Sister Naina
Bangalore, India

Welts From Pressure/Itching

My client was diagnosed with dermagraphism/dermatographic urticaria (a form of hives), which is basically a condition with huge welts that are produced when pressure/itching is applied to the skin. This condition affects 4-5% of the population, and mys-teriously comes and goes with no known cause or cure. It has something to do with an abnormal response of the immune system to pressure on the skin. I tested this patient with NST and treated her for ISM, histamine, leukotrienes, heparin, and IgE and IgM.

In the meantime, I had another client with unusual itching, and on a hunch tested her as if she had dermagraphism, even though she had no welts when she scatched her skin. After testing with NST, I treated her for the same items as the first client (inter-esting). Today, I saw this client, and her uncontrollable, unbear-

able nightly itching has finally been resolved. She has only some itching during the day, which QRT shows is caused by other things we already knew about and were in the process of treating.

When I see the first client again next week, I will find out how she is doing. I asked her to call if her symptoms continued and I have not heard from her since the treatment a few weeks ago.

NAET® Specialist: Debra Lowe, B.A., D.Ac.
Ottowa, Ontario, Canada

Infectious Blisters (Impetigo)

I was sitting right on top of the improvements, and they were there.... and very fast. I will tell my experience of what you did for my little girl. I hadn't heard before of impetigo, so I went searching on the internet to find out what impetigo was. Okay, it was scary to find out. In searching further, I came on your website. Because I don't like medicines so much, I called you immediately. We could come pretty fast. Friday morning we went to Egmond, and I believe that we were in there for at least an hour. It would have been worth three hours for me, because the following day I saw only one spot on her face, and the one on her finger was drying up. It all looked more relaxed. Sunday I say that it looked better in her nose, and you saw her nose, that was pretty bad. Monday it was almost all gone. I am very happy that I found you through the internet, otherwise my daughter would still have the impetigo. Everybody should do NAET® instead of medicines. It may cost you some money, but you get a lot in return and no chemical stuff in your body. Thanks Linda, also from my daughter. Regards, Erika

NAET® Specialist: Linda Menkhorst
Holland, the Netherlands

More on Impetigo...

I treated 10 children for severe impetigo in a week. These children were on antibiotics; seven of them were on their second course of antibiotic treatment. They did not respond to antibiotics. All of them responded well to NAET®: in three treatments, their symptoms got better. I treated these children for Staphylococcus *bacteria,* Streptococcus *bacteria, and in combination with skin. Two of them needed only one treatment, and others needed all three. They all were back to normal in a week.*

NAET® Specialist: Linda Menkhorst
Holland, the Netherlands

NAET® SUCCESS WITH VARIOUS ALLERGENS

Allergy to Cotton Gloves

After 27 years of private practice as a dental hygienist, my hands were breaking out from my gloves within 30 seconds of putting on them (even though I wore cotton gloves). I reacted by redness, itching, blisters, and runny nose. A year and a half ago, I was introduced to NAET®. After my first Basic allergen treatments, I was treated for gloves two times because I did not pass it the first time. After the second treatment I became free of my previous reactions. I could comfortably wear my gloves for eight hours without itching, redness, pimples (blisters), itchy eyes, or runny nose. Thank you NAET®!

NAET® Specialist: Beth Phillips, B.S., R.D.H., R.T., C.N.H.
Minneapolis, Minnesota, U.S.A.

Allergy to Hand Soap

An eight-year-old boy came to the office with a problem with the skin on his fingers. The skin, especially around the nails, was bumpy, wart-like, and was black in color.

Using muscle testing, we determined this was being caused by an allergy to some chemical he was contacting at school. Further questioning revealed that it was the hand soap in the restroom at school.

We treated him for the hand soap, and when I went in to check him after the 20-minute resting period, I examined his fingers again and the blackness was already gone. The skin was still bumpy, but it was now a normal flesh color.

His mother said it was literally disappearing before her eyes. Within a couple of hours his skin became completely normal, and his problem did not return.

NAET® Specialist: Sue Anderson, D.C.
Ann Arbor, Michigan, U.S.A.

Allergy to Pesticides Caused His Hives!

My 19-year-old patient, who is a gardener, had fantastic results from the NAET® treatment for pesticides. His fatigue, lethargy, and insomnia improved dramatically, and hives disappeared completely 48 hours after treatment with NAET® for Malathion®. He has stayed that way for the past year.

NAET® Specialist: Marilyn Chernoff, N.D., Ph.D., M.Ed.
Albuquerque, New Mexico, U.S.A.

NAET® Is Great for Allergies of Any Kind!

I am now retired, but after practicing psychiatry for over 40 years, I must say that I have been pleasantly surprised at the dramatic results that had occurred in my practice over the past 10 years. This has been especially true with pediatric patients.

I had seen a little girl who developed a bad rash on her buttocks every time she sat on her potty chair, who obtained immediate relief when her allergy to plastic was cleared. A four-year-old girl had bad stomach-aches after ingesting milk, but after NAET®

treatments for Basic allergens plus milk mix she told her mother "my stomach doesn't hurt now". A couple of teenage boys had been plagued with multiple asthmatic episodes, but after each received a series of NAET® treatments, they went on to have many months with no serious episodes.

Another young girl was not able to play outdoors without developing severe eczema, but after NAET® treatments for radiation, she was able to play outdoors with no problems. A twenty-month old girl had never stood or walked on her own, but she had successful surgery on both feet at age six months. After receiving NAET® treatment for anesthesia, she stood alone for the first time several hours later, and was walking alone two days later. A six-week old boy had a rash on his face and was very irritable every time he nursed. He received NAET® treatment for his mother's breast milk, then was more content immediately after he resumed nursing, and his rash disappeared within a few days.

These types of dramatic results, along with elimination of specific food allergies, make NAET® stand out, in my opinion, as more effective than any other treatment program that has been developed up to this time in the history of mankind.

NAET® Specialist: Robert M. Prince, M.D.
Charlotte, North Carolina, U.S.A.

Glossary

Acetaldehyde: An aldehyde found in cigarette smoke, vehicle exhaust, and smog. It is a metabolic product of *Candida albicans* and is synthesized from alcohol in the liver.

Acid: Any compound capable of releasing a hydrogen ion; it will have a pH of less than 7.

Acute: Extremely sharp or severe, as in pain, but can also refer to an illness or reaction that is sudden and intense.

Additive: A substance added in small amounts to foods to alter the food in some way.

Adrenaline: Trademark for preparations of epinephrine, which is a hormone secreted by the adrenal gland. It is used sublingually and by injection to stop allergic reactions.

Aldehyde: A class of organic compounds obtained by oxidation of alcohol. Formaldehyde and acetaldehyde are members of this class of compounds.

Alkaline: Basic, or any substance that accepts a hydrogen ion; its pH will be greater than 7.

Allergenic: Causing or producing an allergic reaction.

Allergen: Any organic or inorganic substance from one's surroundings or from within the body itself that causes an allergic response in an individual. An allergen can cause an IgE antibody mediated or non-IgE mediated response. Some of the commonly known allergens are: pollens, molds, animal dander, food and drinks, chemicals of different kind like the ones found in food, water, inside and outside air, fabrics, cleaning agents, environmental materials, detergent, cosmetics, perfumes, etc., body secretions, bacteria, virus, synthetic materials, fumes of any sort, including pesticide fumes, fumes from cooking, etc., and smog. Emotion such as anger or frustration can also become allergens and cause allergic reactions in people.

Allergic reaction: Adverse, varied symptoms, unique to each person, resulting from the body's response to exposure to an allergen.

Allergy: Attacks by the immune system on harmless or even useful things entering the body. Abnormal responses to substances that are usually well tolerated by most people.

Amino acid: An organic acid that contains an amino (ammonia-like NH3) chemical group; the building blocks that make up all proteins.

Antibody: A protein molecule produced in the body by lymphocytes in response to a perceived harmful foreign or abnormal substance as a defense mechanism to protect the body.

Antigen: Any substance recognized by the immune system that causes the body to produce antibodies; also refers to a concentrated solution of an allergen.

Antihistamine: A chemical that blocks the reaction of histamine that is released by the mast cells and basophils during an allergic reaction. Any substance that slows oxidation, prevents damage from free radicals and results in oxygen sparing.

Assimilate: To incorporate into a system of the body; to transform nutrients into living tissue.

Autoimmune: A condition resulting when the body makes antibodies against its own tissues or fluid. The immune system attacks the body it inhabits, which causes damage or alteration of cell function.

Ayurvedic medicine: The traditional system of medicine in India that uses a holistic approach, emphasizing diet, herbal remedies, exercise, meditation, breathing, and physical therapy.

Blackhead (or **open comedo**): A blocked pore in which the "plug" enlarges and pushes through the surface of the skin. The plug's dark appearance is not due to dirt, but rather to a buildup of melanin, the skin's dark pigment.

Candida albicans: A genus of yeast like fungi normally found in the body. It can multiply and cause infections, allergic reactions or toxicity.

Candidiasis: An overgrowth of *Candida* organisms, which are part of the normal flora of the mouth, skin, intestines and vagina.

Catalyst: A chemical that speeds up a chemical reaction without being consumed or permanently affected in the process.

Cerebral allergy: Mental dysfunction caused by sensitivity to foods, chemicals, environmental substances, or other substances like work materials etc.

Chronic: Of long duration.

Closed comedo (or **whitehead**): If the plug in the follicle stays below the surface of the skin, the lesion is called a closed comedo, or whitehead. These usually appear on the skin as small, whitish bumps.

Comedo (plural – comedones): When dead skin cells mix with sebum and get trapped in the opening of a follicle, this is a comedo — the raw material for every kind of acne lesion. It acts like cork in a bottle, trapping dirt, bacteria and sebum inside the follicle, eventually resulting in an acne lesion.

Comedogenic: Substances that are likely to clog your pores.

Contraceptives: Birth control pills (combinations of estrogen and progesterone) are often prescribed for hormonal acne; the estrogen helps suppress the androgens produced by the ovaries. Currently, just two formulas (Ortho Tri-Cyclen LO® and Estro-Step®) have been approved by the FDA for the treatment of acne, but many formulas are just as effective.

Corticosteroids: Small doses of corticosteroids, like prednisone or dexamethasone, may be used to treat acne. They work by curbing inflammation and suppressing the androgens produced by the adrenal glands. Long-term use of prednisone can cause a stubborn form of acne; corticosteroids are most affective when used in combination with oral contraceptives.

Cortisol: Produced by the adrenal glands in response to stress, the hormone cortisol stimulates the sebaceous glands, triggering the production of extra oil. This increases the incidence of comedones, causing acne breakouts.

Crohn's disease: An intestinal disorder associated with irritable bowel syndrome, inflammation of the bowels and colitis.

Cumulative reaction: A type of reaction caused by an accumulation of allergens in the body.

Cytokine: Immune system's second line of defense. Examples of cytokines are interleukin-2 and gamma-interferon.

Dandruff (seborrheic dermatitis): Persistent flaking, scaling or itching of the scalp. For dandruff sufferers, the natural process of scalp-cell renewal is accelerated when fighting off *P. ovale*, a normal fungus found on every human head. This causes dead cells to slough more quickly, creating the dandruff symptoms.

Dermatitis (or **eczema**): Characterized by a rapidly spreading red rash which may be itchy, blistered, and swollen. Atopic dermatitis is related to asthma and hay fever-type allergies, and is often seen in early childhood. Contact dermatitis is usually caused by contact with irritants (detergents or harsh chemicals) or allergens (substance to which the patient is allergic, like rubber, preservatives or a particular fragrance). Individuals with chronic dermatitis will have a longstanding history of irritation in the affected area or areas; the eyelids, neck, and hands are most commonly affected in adults. Dermatitis may come and go throughout a person's life.

Dermatologic surgery: Surgery to repair or improve the function or cosmetic appearance of skin tissue. Methods include laser surgery, cryosurgery, chemical surgery, aspirational surgery (for scarring) and excisional surgery (for acute cysts or nodules). In cases of severe acne scarring, dermatological surgery can be helpful in improving the appearance of some scars.

Dermis: The second layer of the skin, which serves as a foundation for the epidermis and makes up the principle mass of the skin. This layer produces collagen, elastin and reticulin, the substances that lend structure and support to your largest organ. The dermis also houses nerve endings, blood vessels, oil glands and sweat glands.

Demodex mites: Normal residents of human skin, these microscopic creatures are five times more prevalent in patients with rosacea; they are believed to contribute to irritation and flushing in patients with this condition.

Desensitization: The process of building up body tolerance to allergens by the use of extracts of the allergenic substance.

Detoxification: A variety of methods used to reduce toxic materials accumulated in body tissues.

Disorder: A disturbance of regular or normal functions.

Dust: Dust particles from various sources irritate sensitive individual causing different respiratory problems like asthma, bronchitis, hay-fever like symptoms, sinusitis, and cough.

Dust mites: Microscopic insects that live in dusty areas, pillows, blankets, bedding, carpets, upholstered furniture, drapes, corners of the houses where people neglect to clean regularly.

Eczema: An inflammatory process of the skin resulting from skin allergies causing dry, itchy, crusty, scaly, weepy, blisters or eruptions on the skin. Skin rash frequently caused by allergy.

Edema: Excess fluid accumulation in tissue spaces. It could be localized or generalized.

Electromagnetic: Refers to emissions and interactions of both electric and magnetic components. Magnetism arising from electric charge in motion. This has a definite amount of energy.

Elimination diet: A diet in which common allergenic foods and those suspected of causing allergic symptoms have been temporarily eliminated.

Endogenous: Originating from or due to internal causes.

Epidermal cyst: A sac-like growth in the deeper layers of the skin, filled with a soft whitish material. This substance, which is composed of fatty acids and oils, may have an unpleasant odor. In patients with a history of acne, epidermal cysts may occur on the face, scalp and trunk. They are often permanent; even if the material is extracted, the sac remains and the cyst may return. In these cases the entire cyst sac must be excised to prevent recurrence.

Epidermis: The top layer of the skin, which acts as your body's natural suit of armor. The epidermis is made up of corneocytes (the outermost layer of dead skin cells), melanocytes (which produce melanin, the substance that gives your skin its color), and Langerhan cells (which work with the immune system to help you fight off disease).

Environment: A total of circumstances and/or surroundings in which an organism exists. May be a combination of internal or external influences that can affect an individual.

Environmental illness: A complex set of symptoms caused by adverse reactions of the body to external and internal environments.

Enzyme: A substance, usually protein in nature and formed in living cells, which starts or stops biochemical reactions.

Eosinophil: A type of white blood cell. Eosinophil levels may be high in some cases of allergy or parasitic infestation.

Exogenous: Originating from or due to external causes.

Extract: Treatment dilution of an antigen used in immunotherapy, such as food, chemical, or pollen extract.

Favre-Racouchet Syndrome: A skin condition afflicting men and women over age 50 causing large blackheads around the eyes and on the upper cheeks. Unlike acne blackheads, Favre comedones do not regress if left untreated; they must be surgically extracted or treated with topical retinoids.

"Fight or flight": The activation of the sympathetic branch of the autonomic nervous system, preparing the body to meet a threat or challenge.

Follicle (or **sebaceous follicle**): Also called "pores," these tiny holes house the fine hairs that cover our faces and bodies. Oil glands at the base of each follicle are working to produce sebum, which travels up the hair shaft and out onto the surface of the skin.

Follicular macular atrophy: A form of acne scarring characterized by small, soft white lesions resembling whiteheads that didn't fully develop; they may persist for months or years. This kind of scarring is more likely to occur on the chest or back.

Food grouping: A grouping of foods according to their botanical or biological characteristics.

Free radical: A substance with unpaired electrode, which is attracted to cell membranes and enzymes where it binds and causes damage.

Histamine: A body substance released by mast cells and basophils during allergic reactions, which precipitates allergic symptoms.

Holistic: Refers to the idea that health and wellness depend on a balance between the physical (structural) aspects, physiological (chemical, nutritional, functional) aspects, emotional, and spiritual aspects of a person.

Homeopathic: Refers to giving minute amounts of remedies that in massive doses would produce effects similar to the condition being treated.

Homeostasis: A state of perfect balance in the organism, also called "Yin-yang" balance. The balance of functions and chemical composition within an organism that results from the actions of regulatory systems.

Hormones: Chemical substances that govern the processes of the human body. Androgens, the hormones that cause physical maturation during puberty, stimulate the body's production of oil; these are the hormones implicated in acne.

Hypersensitivity: An acquired reactivity to an antigen that can result in bodily damage upon subsequent exposure to that particular antigen.

Hypoallergenic: Refers to products formulated to contain the minimum possible allergens and some people with few allergies can tolerate them well. Severely allergic people can still react to these items.

Ice-pick scars: Most often found on the cheek, ice-pick scars are usually small but deep, with a jagged edge and steep sides. Over time, ice-pick scars may evolve into depressed fibrotic scars. These also have sharp edges and steep sides, but are larger and firm at the base.

Inflammatory: A word that means "causing inflammation." In acne, "inflammatory" is usually used to describe lesions that are inflamed by chemical reactions or bacteria in clogged follicles.

Isopropyl alcohol: A common ingredient of many facial toners, isopropyl alcohol is a strong astringent that can strip the skin of necessary oils, leaving it dry and irritated.

Isotretinoin (Accutane®). The "big gun" in acne therapy, Accutane is used to treat severe inflammatory acne when other treatments fail. The drug reduces sebum production by as much as 85–90% and has a high rate of success for improving acne.

IgA: Immunoglobulin A, an antibody found in secretions associated with mucous membranes.

IgD: Immunoglobulin D, an antibody found on the surface of B-cells.

IgE: Immunoglobulin E, an antibody responsible for immediate hypersensitivity and skin reactions.

IgG: Immunoglobulin G, also known as gammaglobulin, the major antibody in the blood that protects against bacteria and viruses.

IgM: Immunoglobulin M, the first antibody to appear during an immune response.

Immune system: The body's defense system, composed of specialized cells, organs, and body fluids. It has the ability to locate, neutralize, metabolize and eliminate unwanted or foreign substances.

Immunocompromised: A person whose immune system has been damaged or stressed and is not functioning properly.

Immunity: Inherited, acquired, or induced state of being, able to resist a particular antigen by producing antibodies to counteract it. A unique mechanism of the organism to protect and maintain its body against adversity by its surroundings.

Inflammation: The reaction of tissues to injury from trauma, infection, or irritating substances. Affected tissue can be hot, reddened, swollen, and tender.

Inhalant: Any airborne substance small enough to be inhaled into the lungs; e.g., pollen, dust, mold, animal danders, perfume, smoke, and smell from chemical compounds.

Intradermal: method of testing in which a measured amount of antigen is injected between the top layers of the skin.

Keloid: A type of hereditary scarring that occurs more frequently in African-American, Asian and Latino populations. Keloid scarring occurs when the skin cells respond to injury by producing an excess of collagen, which forms into lumpy fibrous masses. These scars appear firm and shiny, and may persist for years.

Keratosis pilaris: Patches of tiny, red, kernel-hard bumps on the cheeks, chest, backs of the arms, shoulders, buttocks and the front of the thighs. Most commonly found in teenagers, keratosis pilaris occurs when hair follicles become clogged with dead skin cells that are not properly sloughed off. It is usually painless and feels spiny to the touch.

Kinesiology: Science of movement of the muscles.

Lipids: Fats and oils that are insoluble in water. Oils are liquids in room temperature and fats are solid.

Lymph: A clear, watery, alkaline body fluid found in the lymph vessels and tissue spaces. Contains mostly white blood cells.

Lymphocyte: A type of white blood cell, usually classified as T-cells or B-cells.

Macrophage: A white blood cell that kills and ingests microorganisms and other body cells.

Mast cells: Large cells containing histamine, found in mucous membranes and skin cells. The histamine in these cells are released during certain allergic reactions.

Mediated: Serving as the vehicle to bring about a phenomenon, e.g., an IgE-mediated reaction is one in which IgE changes cause the symptoms and the reaction to proceed.

Macule: The flat, reddish spots that are the final stage of an acne lesion. Macules may last for up to six months (longer with prolonged sun exposure) but usually leave no permanent scar.

Malignant: A tumor that is out of control, able to invade and destroy nearby tissue.

Melasma (or **cholasma**): Localized hyperpigmentation (brownish blotches) that appear most commonly in women who are pregnant or taking oral contraceptives. These are worsened by exposure to the sun, and can be treated with topical bleaching agents. Rarely, women who are neither pregnant nor taking birth control pills — and occasionally men — may get melasma.

Microcomedo: The first stage of comedo formation; a comedo so small that it can be seen only with a microscope.

Milia: Tiny cysts found mostly in the area around the eyes. They are hard to the touch and deep in the skin. Milia may last for weeks or even months; if they are particularly troublesome to you, consult your dermatologist for professional, safe removal.

Metabolism: Complex chemical and electrical processes in living cells by which energy is produced and life is maintained. New material is assimilated for growth, repair, and replacement of tissues. Waste products are excreted.

Mineral: An inorganic substance. The major minerals in the body are calcium, phosphorus, potassium, sulfur, sodium, chloride, and magnesium.

NAR Foundation: Nambudripad's Allergy Research Foundation, a nonprofit research foundation dedicated to conduct research in allergy elimination of food, chemicals, environmental and other substances using NAET®

NAET® (Nambudripad's Allergy Elimination Technique): A technique to permanently eliminate allergies towards the treated allergens. Developed by Dr. Devi S. Nambudripad and practiced by more than 8,000 medical practitioners worldwide. This technique is natural, non-invasive, and drug-free. It has been effectively used in treating all types of allergies and problems arising from allergies. It is taught by Dr. Nambudripad in Buena Park, California. to currently licensed medical practitioners. If you are a licensed medical practitioner, interested in learning more about NAET®, or NAET® seminars, please visit the website: www. naet.com.

Nervous system: A network made up of nerve cells, the brain, and the spinal cord, which regulates and coordinates body activities.

Nodule: Large and usually very painful, nodules are inflamed, pus-filled lesions lodged deep within the skin. Nodules develop when the contents of a comedo have spilled into the surrounding skin and the local immune system responds, producing pus. The most severe form of acne lesion, nodules may persist for weeks or months, their contents hardening into a deep cyst. Both nodules and cysts often leave deep scars.

Noncomedogenic: Substance that is not likely to clog the pores.

Noninflammatory: In acne, lesions that are not associated with redness in the skin.

NST (Neuromuscular sensitivity testing): A testing technique based on kinesiology to test allergies by comparing the strength of a muscle or a group of muscles in the presence and absence of the allergen.

NTT (Nambudripad's Testing Techniques): A series of standard diagnostic tests used by NAET® practitioners to detect allergies.

Neurotransmitter: A molecule that transmits electrical and/or chemical messages from nerve cell (neuron) to nerve cell or from nerve cell to muscle, secretory, or organ cells.

Nutrients: Vitamins, minerals, amino acids, fatty acids, and sugar (glucose), which are the raw materials needed by the body to provide energy, effect repairs, and maintain functions.

Organic foods: Foods grown in soil free of chemical fertilizers, and without pesticides, fungicides and herbicides.

Overload: The overpowering of the immune system due to numerous concurrent exposures or to continuous exposure caused by many stresses, including allergens.

Parasite: An organism that depends on another organism (host) for food and shelter, contributing nothing to the survival of the host.

Pathogenic: Capable of causing disease.

Pathology: The scientific study of disease; its cause, processes, structural or functional changes, developments and consequences.

Pathway: The metabolic route used by body systems to facilitate biochemical functions.

Papule: The mildest form of inflammatory acne is the papule, which appears on the skin as a small, firm pink bump. These can be tender to the touch, and are often considered an intermediary step between non-inflammatory and clearly inflammatory lesions.

Papulopustular: A type of acne characterized by the presence of papules and pustules.

Peri-oral dermatitis: Primarily affecting women in their 20s and 30s, this condition is characterized by patches of itchy or tender red spots around the mouth. The skin bordering the lips may appear pale and dry, while the chin, upper lips and cheeks become red, dry and flaky. It can also affect the skin around the nose.

Petrochemical: A chemical derived from petroleum or natural gas.

pH: A scale from 1 to 14 used to measure acidity and alkalinity of solutions. A pH of 1-6 is acidic; a pH of 7 is neutral; a pH of 8-14 is alkaline or basic.

Postnasal drip: The leakage of nasal fluids and mucus down into the back of the throat.

Post-inflammatory hyperpigmentation: A darkening of the skin at the site of a healing acne lesion. Most prevalent in African-American, Asian and Latino populations, these spots can last up to 18 months — but may disappear more quickly if you stay out of the sun.

Propionibacterium acnes: A bacterium (*P. acnes* for short) is a regular resident of all skin types; it's part of the skin's natural sebum maintenance system. Once a follicle is plugged, however, *P. acnes* bacteria multiply rapidly, creating the chemical reaction we know as inflammation in the follicle and surrounding skin.

Pseudofolliculitis barbae: The acne-like breakouts commonly called "shaving bumps." As hairs begin to grow back after shaving, waxing or plucking, they get trapped inside the follicle and cause irritation and swelling. Shaving bumps are more common among people with curly hair.

Puberty: The time of life when a child begins the process of physical maturation. Onset is usually in the early teens and is accompanied by a large increase in hormone production — and acne.

Pustule: Small, round acne lesions that are clearly inflamed and contain visible pus. They may appear red at the base, with a yellowish or whitish center. Pustules do not contain a great deal of bacteria; the inflammation is caused by chemical irritation from sebum components such as fatty free acids.

Prostaglandin: A group of unsaturated, modified fatty acids with regulatory functions.

Radiation: The process of emission, transmission, and absorption of any type of waves or particles of energy, such as light, radio, ultraviolet or X-rays.

Receptor: Special protein structures on cells where hormones, neurotransmitters, and enzymes attach to the cell surface.

Retinoids: Chemically related to Vitamin A, retinoids regulate growth of epithelial cells (skin, lung, and gut) and are often powerful antioxidants and cancer preventing agents. Retinoids are also found in many acne mediations, such as Retin-A and Renova; they help dissolve comedones and encourage normal skin-cell sloughing and renewal.

Rosacea: Found in adults between 30 and 60 years of age, rosacea is an acne-like condition that appears only in areas that are likely to flush when a person is embarrassed, excited or hot — primarily the face, neck and chest. The skin is bumpy, red and oily in appearance, and may also involve papules and pustules.

Rotation diet: A diet in which a particular food and other foods in the same "family" are eaten only once every four to seven days.

Salicylic acid: A mild acid that encourages the sloughing of dead skin cells. It stimulates the peeling of the top layer of skin and the opening of plugged follicles, which helps reestablish the normal skin-cell replacement cycle. For milder acne, salicylic acid helps unclog pores to resolve and prevent lesions.

Sebaceous glands: Oil-producing glands at the base of every sebaceous hair follicle — the tiny holes commonly called pores. Found on the face, neck, back and chest, these follicles are the sites of acne lesions.

Sebum: The oily substance produced by sebaceous glands, composed of cholesterol and free fatty acids. Sebum travels up the hair shaft and is expelled onto the skin's surface, keeping it soft and pliable.

Sloughing ("SLUFF-ing"): Part of the skin's natural renewal process, sloughing is the act of shedding dead skin cells to make room for new ones. When cells die, they travel up the hair follicle and out onto the surface of the skin, where they are gradually rubbed away or released into the environment. Until we reach our early 30s, the sloughing and renewal process takes about 28 days. As we age the process begins to slow; by the time we reach our 40s, complete skin renewal may take more than 50 days.

Soft scars: A type of acne scar with gentle, sloping rolled edges that merge with the surrounding skin. They are usually small, circular or linear in shape, and soft to the touch.

Subcutaneous fat: The bottom layer of your skin is composed primarily of fat cells. This part of your skin acts as an insulator, keeping you warm and protecting underlying tissue from shocks and bumps. It's also the place where your hair begins — each hair follicle all over your body has its roots in the subcutaneous layer.

Sensitivity: An adaptive state in which a person develops a group of adverse symptoms to the environment, either internal or external. Generally refers to non-IgE reactions.

Serotonin: A constituent of blood platelets and other organs that is released during allergic reactions. It also functions as a neurotransmitter in the body.

Sublingual: Under the tongue–method of testing or treatment in which a measured amount of an antigen or extract is administered under the tongue, behind the teeth. Absorption of the substance is rapid in this way.

Supplement: Nutrient material taken in addition to food in order to satisfy extra demands, effect repair, and prevent degeneration of body systems.

Susceptibility: An alternative term used to describe sensitivity.

Symptoms: A recognizable change in a person's physical or mental state, that is different from normal function, sensation, or appearance and may indicate a disorder or disease.

Syndrome: A group of symptoms or signs that, occurring together, produce a pattern typical of a particular disorder.

Synthetic: Made in a laboratory; not normally produced in nature, or may be a copy of a substance made in nature.

Systemic: Affecting the entire body.

Target organ: The particular organ or system in an individual that will be affected most often by allergic reactions to varying substances.

Toxicity: A poisonous, irritating, or injurious effect resulting when a person ingests or produces a substance in excess of his or her tolerance threshold.

White blood cells. White blood cells are your body's "Critical Response Unit." When your body encounters unwanted bacteria, it sends an army of white blood cells to attack the intruders. This process is called chemotaxis or the inflammatory response. In acne, it causes pimples become red, swollen and painful.

Witch hazel. A gentle astringent anti-inflammatory and healing properties. Helps to tighten pores and remove excess oil.

Resources

EDUCATION

Nambudripad's Allergy Elimination Techniques (NAET®)
www.naet.com
Website for more information regarding NAET®

Nambudripad Allergy Research (NAR) Foundation
6714 Beach Blvd.
Buena Park, CA 90621
(714) 523-0800
www.narfnet.org
A Nonprofit foundation dedicated to NAET® research

NAET® Seminars
6714 Beach Blvd.
Buena Park, CA 90621
(714) 523-8900
www.naet.com
(click on "Seminar Info")
NAET® Seminar information

Delta Publishing Company
6714 Beach Blvd.
Buena Park, CA 90621
(714) 523-0800
E-mail: naet@earthlink.net
www.naet.com/PublicWebStore
NAET® books

Jacob Teitelbaum M.D.
(410) 573-5389
www.EndFatigue.com
Bestseller books on
CFS/Fibromyalgia Therapies

PRODUCTS

Janice Corporation
198 US Highway 46
Budd Lake, NJ 07828-3001
(800) 526-4237
www.janices.com
Safe health products

Kenshin Trading Corporation
22353 South Western Ave. Suite 201
Torrance, CA 90501 U.S.A.
800-766-1313, (310) 212-3199
Email: websales@kenshin.com
www.kenshin.com
Herbal supplements

Enzyme Formulations, Inc
6421 Enterprise Lane
Madison, WI 53719
(800) 614-4400
www.enzymeformulations.com
Supplements

Xango/ Sandra Stoltz
1112 Montana Ave. # 123
Santa Monica, CA 90403
(203) 256-1443
E mail: sandra11@optonline.net
www.mymangosteen.com/feelgr8
Xango juice

SERVICES

NAET® Specialist Locator
www.naet.com
(click on "Find a Practitioner")
Search by location or name

Bibliography

Allergens

Lazarou J, Pomeranz BH, Corey PN. Incidence of adverse drug reactions in hospitalized patients. *JAMA*. 1998;279:1200-1205.

Poley GE, Slater JE. Latex allergy. *J Allergy Clin Immunol*. 2000; 105(6):1054-1062.

Rapp DJ. *Allergies and Your Family*, New York, NY: Sterling Publishing Co.; 1980.

Sampson HA. Clinical Practice. Peanut Allergy. *N Engl J Med*. 2002;346 (17):1294-1299.

Sicherer SH, Munoz-Furlong A, Sampson HA. Prevalence of peanut and tree nut allergy in the United States determined by means of a random digit dial telephone survey: a 5-year follow-up study. *J Allergy Clin Immunol*. 2003;112(6):1203-1207.

Sicherer SH, Munoz-Furlong A, Sampson HA. Prevalence of seafood allergy in the United States determined by a random telephone survey. *J Allergy Clin Immunol*. 2004;114(1):159-165.

Smith CW. Electrical environmental influences on the autonomic nervous system. 11th International Symposium on Man and His Environment in Health and Disease, Dallas, Texas, February 25-28, 1993. Available at: http://www.aehf.com/articles/1993symp.html.

Allergy Relief

American Academy of Allergy, Asthma and Immunology (AAAAI). *The Allergy Report: Science Based Findings on the Diagnosis & Treatment of Allergic Disorders*, 1996-2001. Available from: http://www.aaaai.org.

Krohn J, Taylor F, Larson EM, *Allergy Relief and Prevention: A Doctor's Complete Guide to Treatment and Self-Care*, 3rd edition. Vancouver, BC: Hartley & Marks Publishers; 2000.

Nambudripad D. Case Histories from the Author's private practice, 1984-present.

ibid., *Eliminate your Pet's Allergies*. Buena Park, CA: Delta Publishing Company; 2006.

ibid., *Freedom From Chemical Sensitivities*. Buena Park, CA: Delta Publishing Company; 2006.

ibid., *Freedom From Environmental Sensitivities*. Buena Park, CA: Delta Publishing Company; 2005.

ibid., *Living Pain Free*. Buena Park, CA: Delta Publishing Company; 1997.

ibid., *Say Good-bye to ADD and ADHD*, 2nd Edition. Buena Park, CA: Delta Publishing Company; 2007.

ibid., *Say Good-bye to Allergy-related Autism*, 2nd Edition. Buena Park, CA: Delta Publishing Company; 2006.

ibid., *Say Good-bye to Asthma*. Buena Park, CA: Delta Publishing Company; 2003.

ibid., *Say Good-bye to Children's Allergies*. Buena Park, CA: Delta Publishing Company; 2001.

ibid., *Say Good-bye to Headaches*. Buena Park, CA: Delta Publishing Company; 2007.

ibid., *Say Good-bye to Illness*, 3rd. Edition. Buena Park, CA: Delta Publishing Company; 2002.

ibid., *Say Good-bye to Your Allergies*. Buena Park, CA: Delta Publishing Company; 2003.

ibid., *The NAET® Guidebook*, 6th Edition. Buena Park, CA: Delta Publishing Company; 2004.

Novak N. Allergen specific immunotherapy for atopic dermatitis. *Curr Opin Allergy Clin Immunol*. 2007;7(6):542-556.

Randolph TG, Moss RW. *An Alternative Approach to Allergies: the New Field of Clinical Ecology Unravels the Environmental Causes of Mental and Physical Ills*, Revised Edition. New York, NY: Harper Perennial; 1990.

Saito Y. Atopic dermatitis: NAET® Treatment of a Newborn Baby with Atopic Dermatitis, *The Journal of NAET Energetics and Complementary Medicine*. 2005;1(3):209-230.

Allergy Statistics

Australian Bureau of Statistics. 2004-2005 National Health Survey: Summary of Results. 27 Feb 2006. Available at: http://www.abs.gov.au/.

Centers for Disease Control and Prevention (CDC). National Center for Health Statistics. Vital and Health Statistics Series. Available at: http://www.cdc.gov/nchs/fastats/default.htm.

Craig LF, Nawar EW, Division of Health Care Statistics. National Hospital Ambulatory Medical Care Survey: 2004 Emergency Department Summary. *Advance Data.* 2006;372:22 (Table 13). Available at: http://www.cdc.gov/nchs/fastats/allergies.htm.

David BK, Golden MD. Stinging Insect Allergy. *American Family Physician.* 2003;67:2541-2546.

Department of Health [United Kingdom]. Hospital Episode Statistics (HES). Available at: http://www.dh.gov.uk/en/Publicationsandstatistics/Statistics/HospitalEpisodeStatistics/index.htm.

Matsumoto I, Odajima H, Nishima S, et al. Change in prevalence of allergic diseases in primary school children in Fukuoka City for the last fifteen years [PubMed Abstract]. *Arerugi.*1999;48(4):435-442.

National Institute of Allergy and Infectious Diseases [United States]. A-Z Health & Science Topics. Available at: http://www3.niaid.nih.gov/health-science/healthtopics/default.htm.

National Institute of Arthritis and Musculoskeletal and Skin Diseases [United States]. Health Information. Available at: http://www.niams.nih.gov/Health_Info/default.asp.

Pleis JR, Lethbridge-Cejku M. Summary health statistics for U.S. adults: national health interview survey, 2005, National Center for Health Statistics. Vital Health Stat 10(232). 2006. Available at: http://www.cdc.gov/nchs/data/series/sr_10/sr10_232.pdf.

The International Study of Asthma and Allergies in Childhood (ISAAC) Steering Committee. Worldwide variation in prevalence of symptoms of asthma, allergic rhinoconjunctivitis, and atopic eczema: ISAAC. *Lancet.* 1998;351(9111):1225-1232.

Applied Kinesiology

Daniels L, Wothingham C. *Muscle Testing Techniques of Manual Examination*, 3rd Edition. Philadelphia, PA: W.B. Saunders; 1972.

Goodheart, GJ. *Applied Kinesiology Research Manual*, Privately published yearly (1964-1998).

Thie JF, Thie M. *Touch for Health: The Complete Edition*. Marina del Rey, CA: DeVorss & Company; 2005.

Basic Science: Oriental Medicine

Beijing College of Traditional Chinese Medicine. *Essentials of Chinese Acupuncture*, First Edition. Beijing, China: Foreign Language Press; 1980.

Hsu H-Y, Peacher WG, *Chinese Herb Medicine and Therapy*, Centennial, CO: Oriental Healing Arts Institute; 1994.

Hsu H-Y, Hus C-H. *Commonly Used Chinese Herb Formulas with Illustrations*, Centennial, CO: Oriental Healing Arts Institute; 1996

O'Connor J, Bensky D (eds). *Acupuncture, a Comprehensive Text.* Shanghai College of Traditional Chinese Medicine. Vista, CA: Eastland Press; 1981.

Otsuka K. *Natural Healing With Chinese Herbs*, Centennial, CO: Oriental Healing Arts Institute; 1982.

Shima M, *The Medical I Ching: Oracle of the Healer Within*. Boulder, CO: Blue Poppy Press; 1992.

Wiseman N, Ellis A. *Fundamentals of Chinese Medicine (Revised)*, Taos, NM: Paradigm Publications; 1994.

Yeung H-C, *Handbook of Chinese Herb Formulas*. Rosemead, CA: Institute of Chinese Medicine; 2004.

Zong L. *Chinese Internal Medicine.* Lectures at SAMRA University, Los Angeles, California; 1985.

Basic Science: Western Medicine

Beeson PB, McDermott W (eds). *Textbook of Medicine*, 12th edition, Philadelphia, PA: W.B. Saunders Company; 1967.

Cecil RL, Goldman L, Bennett JC (eds). *Cecil Textbook Of Medicine*, 21st edition. Philadelphia, PA: W.B. Saunders Company; 2000.

Gray HFRS, Wolff K, Winkelman R. *Gray's Anatomy of the Human Body*, 36th edition. Philadelphia, PA: W.B. Saunders; 1980.

Guyton AC, Hall JE. *Textbook of Medical Physiology*, 11th edition, Philadelphia, PA: W.B. Saunders; 2005

Hepler OE. *Manual of Clinical Laboratory Methods*, 4th ed. Springfield, IL: Charles C. Thomas, 1965.

Janeway C, Travers P, Walport M, Shlomchik M. *Immunobiology: The Immune System in Health and Disease*, 6th edition, New York, NY: Garland Publishing; 2005.

John DT, Petri WA. *Markell and Voge's Medical Parasitology*, 9th. Edition. Philadelphia, PA: W.B. Saunders Company; 2006.

Sonkoly E, Muller A, Lauerma AI, et al. IL-31: a new link between T cells and pruritus in atopic skin inflammation. *J Allergy Clin Immunol.* 2006;117(2):411-417.

Szeidemann Z, Shanabrough M, Leranth C. Hypothalamic Leu-enkephalin-immunoreactive fibers terminate on calbindin-containing somatospiny cells in the lateral septal area of the rat. *J Comp Neurol.* 1995;358(4): 573-583.

Walsh TJ, Dixon DM. Deep Mycoses. In: Baron S, Peake RC, James DA, et al. (eds). *Medical Microbiology* 4th Edition. Galveston, TX: University of Texas Medical Branch; 1996. Available at: http://www.ncbi.nlm.nih.gov/books/bv.fcgi?rid=mmed.section.4006

Complementary and Alternative Medicine Approaches

Bastyr Center for Natural Health. Health Conditions and Concerns. 2007. Available at: http://bastyrcenter.org/content/category/3/130/186/.

University of Maryland Medical Center (UMMC). Complementary and Alternative Medicine Index (CAM). 2004. Available at: http://www.umm.edu/altmed/.

General Interest

Brownstein D. *The Miracle of Natural Hormones*, 2nd Edition. West Bloomfield, MI: Medical Alternatives Press; 1999.

Northrup C. *Women's Bodies, Women's Wisdom*. New York, NH: Bantam Books; 2006.

Nutrition

Cerrat L. *Does Diet Affect the Immune System?* RN Journal. 1990;53:67-70.

Joshi SS, Kuszynski CA, Bagchi D. The cellular and molecular basis of health benefits of grape seed proanthocyanidin extract. Curr *Pharm Biotechnol.* 2001;2(2):187-200.

Krohn J, Taylor F. *Natural Detoxification*, 2nd Edition. Vancouver, BC: Hartley & Marks; 2000.

Mindell E, Mundis H. *Earl Mindell's New Vitamin Bible*, 4th Edition. New York, NY: Grand Central Publishing; 2004.

Pitchford P. *Healing with Whole Foods: Asian Traditions and Modern Nutrition*, 3rd Edition. Berkeley, CA: North Atlantic Books; 2003.

Skin Conditions: History

Hyde JN. In: Hyde JN. Montgomery FH (eds). *A practical treatise on disease of the skin for the use of students and practitioners*. Philadelphia, PA: Lea and Febiger; 1909:174-175.

Turchin I, Adams S. Skimming the surface: A brief history of skin conditions. *Can Fam Physician.* 2005;51(4):477–478.

Skin Disorders: Acne

Baldwin HE. Systemic therapy for rosacea [review]. *Skin Therapy Lett.* 2007;12(2):1-5,9.

Bevins CL, Liu FT. Rosacea: skin innate immunity gone awry? *Nat Med.* 2007;13(8):904-906.

Kane A, Niang SO, Diagne AC, et al. Epidemiologic, clinical, and therapeutic features of acne in Dakar, Senegal. *Int J Dermatol.* 2007;46(Suppl 1):36-38.

Poli F. Acne on pigmented skin. *Int J Dermatol.* 2007;46(Suppl 1):39-41.

Skin Disorders: Athlete's Foot

James IG, Loria-Kanza Y, Jones TC. Short-duration topical treatment of tinea pedis using terbinafine emulsion gel: results of a dose-ranging clinical trial. *J Dermatolog Treat.* 2007;18(3):163-168.

Skin Disorders: Baldness and Hair Loss

Ellis JA, Stebbing M, Harrap SB. Genetic analysis of male pattern baldness and the 5 alpha-reductase genes. *J Invest Dermatol.* 1998;110(6):849-853.

Ellis JA, Stebbing M, Harrap SB. Polymorphism of the androgen receptor gene is associated with male pattern baldness. *J Invest Dermatol.* 2001;116(3):452-455.

Lee WS, Ro BI, Hong SP, et al. A new classification of pattern hair loss that is universal for men and women: basic and specific (BASP) classification. *J Am Acad Dermatol.* 2007;57(1):37-46.

Norwood OT. Male pattern baldness: classification and incidence. *South Med J.* 1975;68(11):1359-1365.

Skin Disorders: Candidiasis

Crook WG. *The Yeast Connection: A Medical Breakthrough.* New York, NY: Random House Vintage Books; 1986.

Ferris DG, Nyirjesy P, Sobel JD, et al. Over-the-counter antifungal drug misuse associated with patient-diagnosed vulvovaginal candidiasis. *Obstet Gynecol.* 2002;99(3):419-425.

Liguori G, Lucariello A, Colella G, et al. Rapid identification of Candida species in oral rinse solutions by PCR. *J Clin Pathol.* 2007;60(9):1035-1039.

Mishra NN, Prasad T, Sharma N, et al. Pathogenicity and drug resistance in *Candida albicans* and other yeast species. A review. *Acta Microbiol Immunol Hung.* 2007;54(3):201-235.

Raska M, Belakova J, Krupka M, et al. Candidiasis—do we need to fight or to tolerate the *Candida* fungus? [review]. *Folia Microbiol (Praha).* 2007;52(3):297-312.

Skin Disorders: Eczema

Berman K. *Eczema.* MedlinePlus, 2007. Available at: http://www.nlm.nih.gov/medlineplus/ency/article/000853.htm.

Eczema. MedlinePlus, 2007. Available at: http://www.nlm.nih.gov/medlineplus/eczema.html.

Larsen F, Hanikin J. Epidemiology of atopic dermatitis. *Immunol Allergy Clinics NA.* 2002;22:1-25.

Lockshin BN, Brogan B, Billings S. Eczematous dermatitis and prurigo nodularis confined to a Becker's nevus. *Int J Dermatol.* 2006;45(12):1465-1466.

National Institute of Arthritis and Musculoskeletal and Skin Disorders (NIAMS). *What is Atopic Dermatitis?* August 2005. Available at: http://www.niams.nih.gov/Health_Info/Atopic_Dermatitis/atopic_dermatitis_ff.asp.

Rudikoff D, Lebwohl M. Atopic dermatitis. *Lancet.* 1998;351(9117):1715-1721.

Schafer T, Kramer U, Vieluf D, et al. The excess of atopic eczema in East Germany is related to the intrinsic type. *Brit J Dermatol.* 2000;143(5):992-998.

Shono M. Allergic contact dermatitis from luliconazole, *Contact Dermatitis.* 2007;56(5):296-297.

Williams HC (ed.). *Atopic Dermatitis: The Epidemiology, Causes and Prevention of Atopic Eczema,* Nottingham, England: University of Nottingham, 2000. Available at: http://www.cambridge.org/uk/catalogue/catalogue.asp?isbn=0511038399.

Patel AR, Vejjabhinanta V, Nouri K. Clinical pearl: the evaluation of the surface area of small pigmented lesions. *Int J Dermatol.* 2007;46(8):872-874.

Skin Disorders: Psoriasis

Cohen AD, Gilutz H, Henkin Y, et al. Psoriasis and the metabolic syndrome. *Acta Derm Venereol.* 2007;87(6):506-509.

Krueger G, Ellis CN. Psoriasis – recent advances in understanding its pathogenesis and treatment. J Am Acad Dermatol. 2005;53(1 Suppl 1):S94-100.

Macdonald A, Burden AD. Psoriasis: advances in pathophysiology and management. *Postgrad Med J.* 2007;83(985):690-697.

Sanchez-Regana ML, Videla S, Villoria J, et al. Prevalence of fungal involvement in a series of patients with nail psoriasis. *Clin Exp Dermatol.* 2007; Nov 5 [Epub ahead of print].

Index